# Finding Your Third Place

*Building Happier Communities*
*(and Making Great Friends Along the Way)*

Richard Kyte

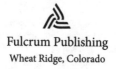

Fulcrum Publishing
Wheat Ridge, Colorado

Library of Congress Cataloging-in-Publication Data
Names: Kyte, Richard, author.
Title: Finding your third place : building happier communities (and making great friends along the way) / Richard Kyte.
Description: Wheat Ridge, Colorado : Fulcrum Publishing, [2024] | Series: The servant leadership series | Includes bibliographical references.
Identifiers: LCCN 2024000248 (print) | LCCN 2024000249 (ebook) | ISBN 9781682754726 (paperback) | ISBN 9781682754733 (ebook)
Subjects: LCSH: Communities--Social aspects. | Sociology. | Interpersonal relations.
Classification: LCC HM756 .K94 2024 (print) | LCC HM756 (ebook) | DDC 307--dc23/eng/20240129
LC record available at https://lccn.loc.gov/2024000248
LC ebook record available at https://lccn.loc.gov/2024000249

Cover design by Kateri Kramer

Unless otherwise noted, all websites cited were current as of the initial edition of this book.

Printed in the United States
0 9 8 7 6 5 4 3 2 1

Fulcrum Publishing
3970 Youngfield Street
Wheat Ridge, Colorado 80033
(800) 992-2908 • (303) 277-1623
www.fulcrumbooks.com

*To my third place "regulars,"*
Tom, Ben, Sam, Ted, and Alcee

# Contents

*God, please send me friends.*

St. Francis of Assisi

# Preface

When I set out a little over a year ago to write a book about third places, I had in mind a straightforward description of social gathering places. I wanted to talk about what they are like, why they are important, and what we can do, as members of communities, to increase their number and accessibility. But writing is like a conversation, and what you start out saying is not always—actually, hardly ever—what you end up saying. As I went about the process of talking to people and reading about third places, I gradually came to see that, first, there were already much better resources addressing practical ways to make our towns and cities more amenable to social connection. Books like Charles Montgomery's *Happy City* and Charles Marohn's *Strong Towns* make a much better argument than I could for the importance of better urban design along with strategies for accomplishing that goal. Second, I came to see that the decline in third places was not due solely to wrongheaded zoning policies and inept urban planning; it was also due to a change in the ways we have come to think and talk about social interaction. We have fewer places to gather than previous generations because we do not value social interaction in the same way, but expressing the problem as one of misguided values is inadequate. It is more complicated than that. What has changed during the past several decades is how we think about our lives, how we think about the nature of friendship, and how we think about the possibilities that come from talking to strangers. We need to discover and then begin deliberately using a more robust and meaningful vocabulary to talk about social connection.

As I asked people why they go to a favorite coffee shop every morning, hang out regularly at a local tavern, belong to a service club, or attend religious services every week in their neighborhood, I came to see that most did not have such a vocabulary. They struggled to articulate why they structured the priorities in their lives the way they did. Few had acted deliberately. Most had instead fallen into a regular pattern by a kind of happy accident: a friend had invited them to join a book club, or they had moved to a new apartment and discovered later that there was a coffee shop they liked just down the block. I talked to people like Dick, who told me he had been attending weekly services at his church for more than forty years. When I asked why, he said, "Well, I wandered in here one day and found the people so friendly and interesting, I just kept coming back."

For most people in previous generations, these kinds of happy accidents were normal. It is the way small groups of people have discovered and learned to spend time together outside of home and work for centuries. But we can no longer count on the circumstances of life to fortuitously lead us into the kind of significant social relationships we require to live full and satisfied lives today. If we wish to live flourishing lives with numerous opportunities for friendship, we must do it deliberately. We must make third places an essential part of the way we think about our lives.

As the theme of this book underwent a transformation, the meaning of the book's title also changed, from something suggesting practical advice about how a person might find a good place to hang out, to discovering a better vision of how to live; that is, finding a way to structure one's life so that one focuses on friendship even more than professional success or the satisfaction of private interests. In short, I came to see that the third place is not just a physical place; it is a metaphor for how one lives in the world, how one might find a place in one's mental geography for cultivating a robust and fulfilling social identity.

# Introduction

*Man is a creature who makes pictures of himself and
then comes to resemble the picture.*

Iris Murdoch, "Metaphysics and Ethics"

I first heard the phrase "third place" in a coffee shop in
Waco, Texas. I was taking a break from a conference
at Baylor University with my friend Beau, a sociology
professor from Centre College. We were discussing the history of coffee shops when he dropped the
phrase "third place." "Wait a minute," I said. "What
is a third place?" Beau mentioned Ray Oldenburg's
books, *The Great Good Place* and *Celebrating the
Third Place*, in which he classifies home as one's first
place, work as one's second place, and the third place
as where one goes to socialize, to make friends.

There are times in your life when you come across
a word or phrase and you think, *I know exactly what
that is, but I don't have a name for it.* The idea of a third
place came at a pivotal time in my life. I was dealing
with a father whose health was in serious decline and

who had become increasingly isolated from both family and friends. At a time when he most needed people in his life, he was turning them away. At the same time, my children were getting older and no longer needed me to go with them to ball games and scouting events. They had their own circles of friends, and I was discovering that much of my social life had been heavily dependent on their activities. Additionally, for the first time in my professional career, I was experiencing burnout. As a result, I was feeling both less productive at work and as if I had no time to do the sorts of activities that would place me in contact with people outside of work. I was beginning to see how easy it would be to slide into a life with less and less room for social interaction. If I did not act deliberately, would I eventually end up like my father, resigned to a life in which grief and regret had settled so deeply as to be inexpressible, a condition described by Emerson as silent melancholy and by Thoreau as quiet desperation?

Learning about third places inspired me to look more carefully at my life. What was I doing to create social connection? Was I doing the work of building relationships today that would help me avoid loneliness as I got older? At the same time, I began integrating Oldenburg's work into a graduate course I was teaching on leadership and community. Over the next several years I made a deliberate effort to reflect more deeply on the significance of third places from the dual perspectives of participant and scholar.

Much has changed in the world since Oldenburg wrote about third places three decades ago. The twin inventions of social media and smartphones have taken over our lives in ways nobody could have imagined at the time, with devastating consequences for the mental health of young people especially. Work has also changed, with many more people working from home or, at least, taking work with them wherever they go—to the coffee shop, to the kitchen table, to their car. The distinction between home and work that defined first and second places has been blurred, and that makes third places even harder to define. Does it even make sense to define types of places by their function when technology has made it possible to do almost anything anywhere?

One thing hasn't changed in the past thirty years, however, and that is the need for human connection. These days there is more appreciation for the depth of that need, and many more social scientists are studying how that need is expressed, satisfied, or frustrated. But we also have more than two thousand years of literature addressing the topic. The centrality of love and friendship in our lives has always been a concern of philosophers, poets, novelists, and dramatists. The need that underlies our longing for third places isn't new; what is new is the challenges technology has presented to us as we try to satisfy that need. In this book, I will rely upon the social sciences, philosophy, literature, and personal stories to show why I think third places are significant. They are a key to cultivating friendship in a world that is increasingly socially fragmented.

For nearly every society in the world's history, as people aged, they became more deeply rooted in their communities, but that is no longer true. A survey conducted a few years ago by OnePoll asked two thousand Americans to answer a series of questions about friendship. They discovered that the average person has not made a new friend in the past five years, and most people's social circle reached its peak in their early twenties. We are the first society to build a world in which the older we get, the more disconnected we become.

For decades we have been designing cities with faster roads, bigger houses, more convenience, and less interaction. We have fallen into an addictive cycle, requiring more and more funds to maintain a vast, aging, and ultimately dysfunctional infrastructure. Then we spend even more money to address the problems created by social isolation: homelessness, depression, drug addiction, and domestic abuse.

The other day I was driving to see some old friends. They live a couple of hours away, and I hadn't been to their house for several years. Approaching the outskirts of town, I saw a large unplanted field. Housing lots were staked out with electrical boxes poking up here and there through the weeds. Another half mile along the road, and I was driving past several huge new apartment complexes on the left. On the right were dozens of houses spaced out on three- and four-acre lots along serpentine roads.

The town is reported to be among the fastest-growing populations in the Midwest, and that certainly seemed true based on the amount of new construction I was seeing. The traffic was greater than the last time I had visited, the parking lots of the apartment buildings were full, and the houses, with their two- and three-car garages, looked prosperous. I could see playground equipment and trampolines in the backyards; boats and campers were sprinkled here and there on the driveways.

Coming into town, the highway was bordered on both sides by gas stations, hotels, banks, fast-food restaurants, and drive-thru coffee shops. Turning right at the second stoplight, I proceeded two blocks until I crossed the old commercial district, where the highway used to run through town before the bypass was constructed in the 1970s. Looking to my right and left as I negotiated the four-way stop, I could see a couple of taverns, a café, and what looked like a gift shop. It was hard to tell how many of the businesses were open. Half a dozen cars could be seen parked along the street. What used to be a thriving commercial district now served as a transition between the old and new sections of town.

I drove another several blocks through neighborhoods with houses of varying shapes, sizes, and conditions, most of them built sometime between 1920 and 1980. Unlike the newer developments on the outskirts of town, this area had little uniformity to it. Every block had its own character. I passed by an elementary school, a couple of churches, and a large park with playgrounds and a ballfield. It was a beautiful summer weekend, and a ballgame was in progress. A few people sat in the stands. Half a dozen children ran around on the nearby playground, the parents standing off to the side visiting with one another. They were the only people I had seen outside talking to one another since I had passed the city limits.

How is it that a person can drive through a prosperous community with a growing population and see so few people socializing? The answer is obvious and regrettable. As a general practice, we no longer build for social connection. We build private spaces, and we build commercial spaces: home and work. We build roads to connect the two. We rarely build for public life. The park where social interaction was taking place was built about seventy-five years earlier.

The neglect of public spaces is a problem because, whether we want to admit it or not, we are dependent on one another, and we can't always count on others to agree with our interests. We need places to work out our thoughts about how to live together. Whether we are talking about a household, a community, or a country, living together well is not just a matter of getting the rules right. It is not just negotiation; it is conversation. That means we need to talk to one another and listen to one another. We must participate in a shared public life.

When people take time to talk to strangers, they frequently discover that they have a great deal in common. They discover that they like the same music, they have similar hobbies, they have had similar childhood experiences, they have the same dreams and hopes. Later, when they go out among a crowd of strangers, they find that their perspective has changed. Instead of a crowd of potential threats, they begin to see others as potential friends.

Our ancestors understood this. Every successful civilization has integrated means by which people can meaningfully interact with one another in public spaces. The ancient Athenians had the agora; the Algonquians had the sacred fire; the English had the pub. They are the places where friendships are formed, where meaning is created, where culture flourishes.

We still have places where people can socialize, but, for the most part, we are no longer building with the specific intention of bringing members of our communities together into shared public spaces. If we don't build for that purpose, we will lose the sense of common ties that bind us together as a people. No effort to teach our children the proper values, the proper history, the proper rules of civic engagement, will make up for that loss.

If you look hard in America, you can still find places where public life is hanging on. You can find places where people from different families and workplaces come together to talk about their shared concerns and interests. In those places, you hear people talk about "our kids," "our schools," "our town," "our home," "our country." But in too many communities, the remnants of public life are hanging on only in places that were built generations ago. The challenge is great because, for a variety of reasons, we don't need public gathering spaces just to survive as previous generations did. Yet we do need gathering places to thrive.

A thriving community is one with abundant resources that are broadly distributed, allowing individuals and groups throughout the community to flourish. A key indicator is how easy it is for children born into families with social or economic disadvantages to become fully functioning, autonomous adults who make meaningful contributions to the lives of others. As we will see, this happens most readily in places that have a variety of robust social connections, allowing opportunities for friendships to form and for residents to interact with and get to know one another.

We have forgotten how to build thriving communities because we have forgotten who we are. We picture our cities as vast, complex machines, designing them for greater productivity and efficiency. But human beings are not machines. We are social animals, and we thrive only when we create conditions suitable for the cultivation of friendship. We need to change the way we picture our lives.

# CHAPTER ONE

# Why Are We Feeling So Bad About Our Lives?

*In mourning it is the world which has become poor and empty; in melancholia it is the ego itself.*

Sigmund Freud, "Mourning and Melancholia"

Here is the puzzle. Most of the objective evidence shows that the world is getting better every decade, and not just a little bit better—much better. Life expectancy is going up around the world; extreme poverty is being reduced; air and water quality are improving; diseases are being treated more widely and effectively. Yet people are feeling much worse about their lives and the condition of the world they are living in.

The skeptics will say, "Wait a minute. What about climate change? What about inequality? What about gun violence? What about plastics in the ocean?" But their objections make the point. All those things are genuine causes for concern. They require serious, urgent attention; however, they aren't significantly more threatening than the crises my parents faced when I was a child.

Crises faced in the past always seem less grave than the ones we face today precisely because they took place in the past. We can see how they have been resolved, but we can't see into the future. We can't be sure the things that threaten catastrophe in the next few years will be diverted. But the point is this. Those who lived through the crises of sixty years ago also didn't know whether the many difficulties facing them could be overcome, but, for some reason, they were not collectively demoralized by the seriousness of the challenges.

I was born in 1962. That is the year of the Cuban Missile Crisis when nuclear holocaust seemed imminent; that is the year Rachel Carson's book *Silent Spring* was published, warning that insecticides were destroying bird life all over the planet; that is the year James Meredith, the first Black student to attend the University of Mississippi, had to be escorted onto campus by US marshals. In December of 1962, the smog in London was so bad that more than three hundred people died in just four days from breathing the air.

Yet my parents' generation was not pessimistic about the world into which I was born. On the contrary, they were determined to make things better.

They built bomb shelters in their backyards and rallied behind a president who would stand up to Khrushchev's nuclear intimidation. They banned DDT and established the Environmental Protection Agency. They passed the Civil Rights Act. Most importantly, they did not despair.

Today, many young people are in despair.

Marriage has been declining steadily over the past fifty years; today the marriage rate is about half of what it was in 1972. And the young couples who have decided to make a life together are more reluctant than past generations to bring children into the world.

Loneliness also seems to be increasing, although researchers do not have reliable data going back very far. The world's largest survey on loneliness, conducted by the BBC in 2018 and involving fifty-five thousand participants, found that one-third of people reported that they often or very often feel lonely. And those numbers are even worse for young people, with 40 percent of those aged between sixteen and twenty-four saying they often or very often feel lonely.

Along with declining emotional well-being for individuals, trust in other people and the institutions upon which we depend has also been falling. In chapter two, we will look more closely at the work of Robert Putnam, the author of *Bowling Alone*, who has documented the decline in social capital and civic engagement since the 1950s.

When Putnam's book was published in 2000, there was a tendency on the part of many observers to blame the decline of social capital on some development in the recent past: some blamed computers, others television and radio, others blamed the growth of suburban housing and the loss of neighborhoods. Today, many point to more recent developments, such as smartphones and social media. As we will see, there is evidence to suggest that the widespread adoption of these new technologies has caused a great deal of psychological harm, especially among young people who are the earliest and heaviest users of them. But it would be a mistake to settle on just one specific cause of collective malaise. The truth is, we are feeling worse about our lives because each generation spends less time doing the things that make us feel good about our lives: forming and tending to loving relationships.

Human beings are social animals. From the time we are born, we tend to flourish when we are enmeshed in a wide network of mutual accountability: nurturing and being nurtured in turn. The longest-running study on human flourishing is the Harvard Study of Adult Development. Researchers connected with the study have been following 724 men since 1938, contacting them every two years to ask questions about their physical and mental health. They recently added about thirteen hundred descendants of the original participants to the study. An immense amount of data has been collected from the study, but one overarching finding stands out: close personal relationships contribute significantly to well-being. But we shouldn't need a study to tell us that. We can see it in our own everyday experiences.

In *Cultivating a Servant Heart*, Caitlin Wilson records an interview with Aaron Rasch, a caregiver for Bubba, a nonverbal man who had spent years in and out of mental institutions. Aaron had been warned that caring for Bubba would be a challenge. At first, it did not go well. Bubba would lash out at Aaron, yelling, throwing dishes, trying to hit or bite him. But then Aaron had an idea. He reached out to Bubba's sister and asked about the things Bubba liked to do. He paid careful attention to Bubba's garbled sounds and gestures. Aaron said, "It took less than a week, and Bubba's incidents became fewer and fewer. From four to five per day to once every couple weeks. It became clear that being understood was something important to Bubba, but not a task expected from caregivers. Listening to Bubba's deeper story gave insight into what every human being wants, to be understood and connected to people we care about."

Bubba's frustration grew out of a universal human need. When our need for connection is not satisfied, we become frustrated, anxious, depressed.

Consider another example. After a recent talk, the mother of a ten-year-old girl came up to me and told me about her frustration with the teachers and administrators at her school. Her daughter, she explained, had some learning difficulties that sometimes resulted in outbursts in the classroom. Teachers found that they could calm her down by taking her into another room and giving her a tablet to work on independently. But this caused her to fall further behind, so when she returned to the classroom, she was lost. This would result in another outburst, followed by time alone with the tablet. The mother finally convinced teachers at the school not to remove her daughter from the class but instead to help her work through her learning difficulties. With the parents and teachers working together, the daughter was finally catching up to her classmates and the outbursts were becoming less frequent.

This story serves as a parable to help us understand what is going on in the world today. Technology (like the tablet) makes it easier to do things by reducing the extent of our dependence on one another. The teachers don't have to deal with the student's outbursts; the student does not have to work through her frustrations with her teachers and classmates. But the technology has a price. By reducing mutual dependence, the student becomes less a part of the group. She no longer belongs with them, no longer feels needed or loved.

There are exceptions, of course. Text-to-speech software helps people with visual impairments read printed text. Sip-and-puff systems allow those who who are paralyzed or lack sufficient fine motor skills to control devices like joysticks or switches. In numerous cases like these, technology can be used to help people connect, to facilitate belonging. But such uses of technological innovations, while significant, are the exception, not the rule.

The overall effect of advances in technology is to lessen our dependence on one another, which inevitably results in a weakening of ties throughout society. Whether we are talking about a smartphone, a car, or a washing machine, most forms of technology increase our power and freedom. They provide us with the ability to do more and the ability to do it more conveniently. Both the power and the freedom that technology provides reduce our mutual dependence, and some forms of technology do this much more extensively than others. It is the price we pay for all the improvements in quality of life mentioned earlier—like increased life expectancy and reduction of diseases. Most of us would not want to live in a world without the benefits of technology.

As our dependency on one another decreases, we change the ways in which we live and work in relation to one another. The invention of the auto-mobile makes it easier for people to work in places miles away from where they live; the computer makes it possible to work and interact with people anywhere in the world. Power and freedom. Yet, if we aren't careful, we can end up living in ways that make us feel miserable, even as we get more of what we want.

An example is a story I heard from an engi-neer who was working for an organization in Africa to provide safe drinking water for rural villages. His organization wanted to reduce the incidence of disease from contaminated water supplies while also lessening the burden on women who had to spend much of their days carrying water from distant springs. One of the results, they expected, would be that girls would be able to stay in school longer, since they wouldn't be needed to carry water for the family. After placing wells in sev-eral villages, the engineer returned months later to find that not everyone was happy. The new water source had indeed reduced the incidence of disease, and more girls were now staying in school to further their edu-cation. But the wells also had an unanticipated effect: many of the women who had spent a good part of each day walking and talking with one another were now spending the entire day in their homes doing household chores alone. The women had lost their chief means of social connection, and the villages had lost much of their joy and vitality.

Why couldn't they have both clean water and social connection? Well, they probably could, but the patriarchal social structure of the villages was slow to change. This is one of the problems with technological developments. They can change the ways we interact with one another very quickly, sometimes in a day, or a few weeks, or months. But the social structures we have developed to manage our lives together were shaped over decades or even centuries. They can be hard to reshape, and we often do not know how—or cannot agree on how—to reshape them quickly and effectively.

An example of this in our own country is the crisis of homelessness, which is afflicting many large to mid-size cities. We have always had people who struggled with mental illness or addiction, people who could not find a job or manage to earn enough to pay for basic necessities. So why is homelessness today a much bigger social issue than it was, say, thirty or forty years ago?

There are many contributing factors, including an undersupply of housing resulting from short-sighted

development strategies and misguided zoning policies. But an even greater contributor to the problem
is the fact that we have many fewer communities of
the sort that those in need can rely upon to help them
out. The past century of steady technological progress means that those who have the good fortune to
grow up in a relatively stable home and who enjoy
good health and economic stability are able to live relatively free from obligations to others. They are able
to provide for themselves and those closest to them
without needing much help. But this means they are
not part of a network of mutual dependency. They are
not readily available to provide support for those who
do not have the same advantages.

Highly educated professionals tend to have
larger and nicer homes, more disposable income, and
much more freedom to act independently than the
rest of the population. As a class, they are also much
less likely to be active members of churches or other
organizations with a prosocial mission. They tend to
group together. They live in the same neighborhoods,
work in the same buildings, and vacation in the same
places as other members of their class. This means
we have many more communities composed almost
entirely of people with relatively low levels of need. At
the same time, we have more communities composed
almost entirely of people with particular kinds of

needs: retirement communities, for example. While residents of these places have relatively high levels of need, they also have the means to address those needs proactively without burdening others. The end result is that we have fewer communities made up of people with varying levels of need and resources. So, where do those people go who, for one reason or another, cannot live without the assistance of others and do not have the resources to fulfill their needs on their own? They are pushed from one place to another until they end up together, in shelters or tent cities or under bridges—entire populations of people who in a less technologically advanced society would be widely distributed throughout many different communities composed of people who routinely helped one another as a matter of course.

This situation isn't anyone's fault. It is human nature to want a better life—a life in which one can pursue the kinds of activities and lifestyle in which one hopes to find fulfillment, among the people with whom one feels comfortable and at ease. The difference today as compared to earlier times in the world's history is that so many more people have the ability to do that. And those who do not have the ability are worse off for it.

Actually, we are all worse off for it. One of the arguments of this book is that caring for one another is a source of significant meaning in life—those with more ability and greater resources entering into relationships with those who have less ability and fewer resources. And this is why life in nations with greater economic means and a higher level of technological development increasingly seems shallow or superficial. It is one of the reasons we have so many people writing books about topics like "authenticity" and "mindfulness," reminding us that authenticity is found in joining together in purposeful action or that the peace of mind we long for is found in acts of loving attention. We sense a lack of depth in our lives but aren't sure what to do about it. We try to fill our lives up by adding things to our bucket lists, not realizing our bucket has a hole in it.

In addition to the fact that technology in general makes us less dependent on one another and therefore less socially connected, there are certain forms of technology that do not just incidentally make our lives worse, they are designed to do just that. I'm thinking here of smartphones and social media. If we are going to live in a world that makes use of the many quality-of-life improvements that technology affords us while also minimizing its isolating effects, it is going to be very important that we distinguish between technology that has incidental negative effects and technology that has negative effects because it is doing just what it has been designed to do.

The problem with social media use among teens is threefold: it interferes with the reward system of the brain, it focuses attention on image-based status that is always subject to the whims of an audience, and finally, it diminishes time that could otherwise be spent in face-to-face interactions, which are more likely to help young people develop an enduring sense of self-worth. When you pair this with an online culture that is highly judgmental and censorious rather than loving and forgiving, you have a recipe for collective depression. The important thing to note is that most of these adverse effects do not come from "problems" that can be designed out of social media programs. They arise from social media functioning exactly the way it is supposed to.

Imagine a pharmaceutical company announcing plans to market a new medical device to children. The device would inject tiny amounts of dopamine into kids' brains every few minutes, making them happier throughout the day. If a researcher at a medical institution or university proposed an experiment of this kind, it would be rejected at once. Most parents, of course, would never stand to have their children experimented upon in this way. But the proposal would also have to pass a review board overseeing research on human subjects to ensure they are not exposed to undue risks. Such boards are especially rigorous when it comes to protecting children. Yet, social media companies employ neuroscientists who carefully study, measure, and conduct experiments on the ways its products affect the brain. Their programmers create algorithms that are designed to keep users scrolling on their phones by triggering the release of dopamine. The more the user anticipates a positive response, the better they feel.

According to a recent report by the US surgeon general Dr. Vivek H. Murthy, social media is a significant contributor to mental health decline among the nation's youth. The report states that "frequent social media use may be associated with distinct changes in the developing brain in the amygdala (important for emotional learning and behavior) and the prefrontal cortex (important for impulse control, emotional regulation, and moderating social behavior), and could increase sensitivity to social rewards and punishments." And yet, there is no suggestion that we treat social media like an untested drug or an environmental toxin.

The situation regarding social media today is comparable to that with lead poisoning fifty years ago. We know it is probably bad for kids in all kinds of ways, but we don't have absolute proof, and there are so many desirable uses for it, and so much money to be made from it, we seem content to just wait and see. In short, social media companies are conducting a vast experiment on the developing brains of our nation's children, and we may not know the full extent of the impacts until it is too late to reverse them.

But the problem is not just social media, it is also the technology most widely used to access social media. In the United States today, approximately 97 percent of American teens have their own cell phones, and they use them constantly. A report from Common Sense Media revealed that in 2021, tweens and teens (eight to eighteen years old) spent an average of eight hours and thirty-nine minutes a day in front of a screen. Children from middle- and lower-income households spent about two hours a day more on screens than children from higher-income households. We are raising a generation of children who are more disengaged from the world around them than any generation in history. It doesn't matter whether they are using social media, texting, or playing games on their phones. While their minds are occupied by what's on the screen they are not attending to the real world.

Having a cell phone means we do not have to look for landmarks or stop and ask for directions when we are traveling. We don't have to ask a stranger for advice or notice what is happening with the weather. They allow us to be more self-sufficient but also less capable at the same time. We can have connections to more people but less ability to engage them in mean-ingful conversation. They make our lives both busier and lonelier, more informed and less competent.

New technology tends to raise new ethical ques-tions because it changes how humans interact with one another and the rest of the world. For example, one of the indirect consequences that nobody could have foreseen was that widespread use of cell phones would reduce the amount of empathy people have for one another. That is the surprising development reported by Sherry Turkle in her book, *Reclaiming Conversation: The Power of Talk in a Digital Age*.

Speaking of her work with a middle school in upstate New York, Turkle notes: "As the . . . middle schoolers began to spend more time texting, they lost practice in face-to-face talk. That means lost practice in the empathic arts—learning to make eye contact, to listen, and to attend to others."[1] The problem is this: human beings do not simply interact with the world, they are also shaped by their interaction. This interac-tion continues to shape us throughout our lives, often in ways we do not realize.

Technology that gives us more freedom and control is in many ways good. It helps us be more effi-cient, be safer, stay healthier, and be more informed. But there is an old saying: "Be careful what you wish for, you might get it." Turkle quotes a sixteen-year-old talking about his experience with gaming: "On computers, if things are unpredictable, it's in a predictable way." Then she observes, "Real people, with their unpredictable ways, can seem difficult to contend with after one has spent a stretch in simulation."[2]

An important ethical lesson parents teach their children is how to get along with other people—most importantly, how to treat people as people (with kindness and respect) and not as objects to be manipulated. Most major ethical lapses come from a failure to learn or remember this lesson. It requires virtues like patience and acceptance to set one's own desires aside because other people may be harmed or inconvenienced by them. If a person's will is not formed by the contingencies of the real world—that is the obstacles and impediments to one's desires—then a new kind of frustration appears: a frustration born out of an inarticulate desire for the world to be other than it is, but without knowing how to bring it into being with others' consent.

The most profound influence on our lives comes from the fact that the world we live in does not respond to our wishes. That fact means that most of our daily behavior is conditioned by the need to continually adjust ourselves to an often undesirable set of circumstances: it is raining, it is too hot outside, the milk in the refrigerator went sour, the grocery store is five miles away, the person I like doesn't like me. Virtual reality lessens the brute resistance of the world as the central defining feature of human existence; in doing so, it obscures our relationship to the world and to other people.

When it comes to the dangers that threaten our bodies, we eventually realize the threats and do our best to address them. Our need for things like water, food, security, and health are tied directly to universal perceptions of pleasure and pain. If our water is contaminated and we are unable to drink it, we suffer from thirst. If we do not have food, we become hungry. Our natural desire corresponds to that which our bodies need. But what happens when we lack beauty in our surroundings? What happens when our lives lack purpose? What happens when we do not have any friends?

When the human need for mental or spiritual well-being goes unmet, we tend not to experience the symptoms as something directly connected to the need. Young men who are lonely do not immediately reach out toward potential friends the way someone suffering from thirst reaches out for water. Instead, they tend to become angry and aggressive. In fact, the rise of phenomena like hate crimes and toxic masculinity likely have more to do with increasing isolation than with the spread of dangerous ideas. Yet, the response to those who express hatred of others is often to shame or shun, thus deepening the loss that led to expressions of hatred in the first place.

Consider the rising amount of anxiety throughout the nation. In 2022, the US Preventive Services Task Force, an advisory panel that provides healthcare screening guidelines, recommended that all adults under age sixty-five be screened for anxiety. Early in 2023, they recommended anxiety screening for youth. According to the National Survey on Drug Use and Health, anxiety increased from 8 percent in 2008 to nearly 15 percent in 2018 among eighteen-to-twenty-five-year-olds.

Our response to this rise has been to treat anxiety as a significant and urgent health problem by emphasizing the need to diagnose cases earlier so they can be treated. The catch is that behavioral health is woefully underfunded, and providers are overburdened. Counseling services in most schools and universities have reached their limit. When students are referred to outside services, they often find themselves on a months' long waiting list for an initial visit.

The more one studies the situation, the more it looks like increasing screening and hiring more therapists is a losing game. It's like bailing water out of a sinking boat. At some point, you have to fix the leak. The big question is: What is causing the rising rates of anxiety? If you ask those who are experiencing anxiety, they point to things going on in their lives or out in the world, like discrimination, harassment, trauma, health, safety, finances, and politics. Therapists are even coming up with new names to describe common forms of anxiety based on the objects of patients' concern. Thus, we get new terms, like "eco-anxiety," based on severe worries about our environmental future. But, as we have seen, people have always faced severe difficulties, and it's simply not true that things are objectively worse today than they were for previous generations. Could it be that there are deeper causes for anxiety than what people experiencing it report?

Perhaps we should look at the ways we think about things instead of the things themselves. What if the reason for rising rates of anxiety is not that things are getting worse but that we are getting worse at thinking about things in constructive ways? A study published in the *Proceedings of the National Academy of Sciences* reported that cognitive distortions—patterns of thinking associated with anxiety and depression—have surged in the last few decades. The authors speculate that our society may be undergoing a collective depression.

Anxiety does not happen just because there are stressors in a person's life. Anxiety is what is known in psychology as an internalizing disorder. There is a fault in the way one processes incidents, and that results in various forms of distress, from worry and fear to episodes of insomnia and panic attacks. The best way to deal with an internalizing disorder is through the cultivation of mental discipline, but that takes time and practice. A person who spends years cultivating a self-image that depends on things turning out the right way and people seeing them the way they want them to shouldn't be surprised when their lives fall apart. All the king's therapists and all the king's counselors won't put them back together again.

At one point in time, it was assumed that developing mental discipline was an essential part of education. That is, after all, why the various branches of academic study are known as "disciplines." But in recent decades two things have happened. First, our educational system has elevated STEM (science, technology, engineering, and math) fields and professional studies like health care, business, law, and education. What they all have in common is learning how to manipulate and transform the outside world. At the same time, the areas of study that traditionally taught young people how to develop internal discipline—like philosophy, religion, literature, and the arts—have been declining and changing their focus. Increasingly, the humanities seek to maintain relevance by focusing on subjects like "applied ethics," "cultural studies," "women's studies," and "professional writing," most of which have an external focus. The result is that we are gradually getting better and better at transforming the world outside our heads while at the same time we are getting worse and worse at controlling the thoughts going on inside them.

One sign that we are losing control of our minds is the fact that wellness is now a $4 trillion industry. People know something is wrong and are grasping at solutions. The marketplace is happy to provide those solutions in the form of essential oils, biohacking, facial exercises, fitness apps, yoga classes, and detox regimens. It's not that any of these things are bad, it's just that they don't address the root of the problem. Exercising, for example, will certainly make a person feel better, but it won't fundamentally change the way one thinks about things.

The problem, as the Stoic philosopher Epictetus pointed out nearly two thousand years ago, is that the more we focus on changing the world around us to make us feel better, the more we feel emotionally tethered to it. If our emotional life is bound too closely to the circumstances outside our heads, then no matter how much better we make things, we will always feel as if we don't have control over our lives.

There will always be a small percentage of people who experience severe forms of anxiety and need therapy to help them cope with their affliction. But when we see a huge increase in anxiety levels across the population in a relatively short period of time, that's a clue that something is seriously wrong. It is likely that the reason anxiety is increasing so rapidly is not simply a response to what is happening in the world but also changes in the ways we think about what is happening. Fortunately, that's something we can control, and we have centuries of wisdom to help us do that better. We just have to turn once again to the sources that can help us think more clearly about human relationships.

The great challenge of our time is learning how to make use of the many technological advances that improve the quality of life without allowing those same advances to undermine our connection to one another—connections that are every bit as essential to human flourishing as food, water, shelter, and security. Aristotle argued that society precedes the individual. He said, "Anyone who cannot form a community with others, or who does not need to because he is self-sufficient, is no part of a city-state—he is either a beast or a god."[3] It is only in society that we learn the virtues, the character traits that allow us to flourish. It is in society that we learn patience, courage, generosity, justice, and love. It is in society—that is, in a robust network of mutual accountability—that we learn to be human.

But can we meet that challenge? Can we develop new social structures that allow us to form deep and meaningful connections to others even when we do not need to in order to survive? Can we reinvent forms of life that allow us to flourish together? I do not know the answer to those questions, but I know we must try. We must try to do something deliberately and intentionally that previous generations of human beings did out of necessity. We must create places for the purpose of deepening our connections to others; not private places set aside from the rest of humanity; not workplaces where we go to earn a living, but a different kind of place. A third place.

# CHAPTER TWO

# Revisiting the Third Place

*There is nothing which has yet been
contrived by man, by which so much happiness
is produced as by a good tavern or inn.*

James Boswell, *The Life of Samuel Johnson*

When Ray Oldenburg first wrote about third places in *The Great Good Place* in 1989, online communities were still more than a decade away. At the time, there were only a few computer-based discussion forums like Usenet and Compuserve's CB Simulator, populated almost entirely by a handful of diehard computer enthusiasts. It was not until the early 2000s that social media companies like Friendster, LinkedIn, MySpace, and Facebook became popular with the wider public and began to permanently alter the social landscape. Yet, even in 1989, Oldenburg's work had an air of nostalgia about it. He was writing about appreciating and preserving something that was being lost.

The nostalgic feeling about third places is evident to anyone who watches an episode of *Cheers*, the popular television series that aired for eleven seasons beginning in 1982. The theme song, "Where Everybody Knows Your Name," written by Gary Portnoy and Judy Hart-Angelo, has a plaintive sound to it—as if the place where everybody knows your name is a place remembered or imagined or longed for. It's not the place where you are, or where you typically go; it's the place where "sometimes you want to go"; it's the place where you would "like to get away" from the troubles of the world. It is a mark of how successfully the program captured our longing for regular social connection, and how atrophied the possibilities for connection are today, that *Cheers* is still regarded as a prototypical third place, even among those who were born well after the series ended.

But third places are not remnants of a bygone age. They are just rarer than they used to be, and that is why it is important to look more closely at them. What are they like? What social function do they serve? Under what conditions do they thrive? How can we make them part of our lives? The first step is simply recognizing what a third place is, and for this, there is no better source than Oldenburg himself, who describes their characteristics.

The first characteristic is that third places are **neutral ground**. People are free to come and go, and nobody has the responsibilities of the host or the obligations of the guest. This fact creates conditions in which **people can meet as equals**, which is the second characteristic of third places. People who occupy very different social or professional roles find it quite natural to come together in third places. This makes it very different from the workplace, which is generally hierarchical in structure. Whereas status tends to be emphasized in the workplace, it is irrelevant in third places. What matters more is personality. This lack of status means third places tend to be inclusive: anybody can speak up; anybody can direct the flow of conversation. The agenda is always in the room; that is, what people talk about are the things that are on their minds, not what just one person thinks is important. As a result, such places are animated by **lively conversation**, which is the third characteristic. Storytelling, joking, and playful banter are the norm.

Yet another characteristic of third places is their **accessibility**. They are easy to get to and one can count on them being open. They are the type of place one is free to just drop in at any time. They don't require planning or appointments or a great deal of travel.

The fifth characteristic is that there are "**regulars**" who show up consistently and give a place its unique personality. This personality comes from the people who inhabit the place and from their friendly relations with one another. A coffee shop inhabited by individuals silently engrossed in their phones or laptops is no more a third place than a large public restroom with several stalls.

Another, perhaps incidental, characteristic, is that third places tend to be rather **ordinary**. They are not unusually expensive or fashionable but have a predictably low profile. The latest trendy restaurant that everybody wants to check out is not a third place. What draws people to third places is not their aesthetics but rather another characteristic—their **playful mood**. Hearing regular, genuine laughter is one of the surest signs you have stepped into a third place.

The final characteristic is that the place feels like a "**home away from home**." It is a place one can go, not to see and be seen, but to relax and feel welcome. A third place is comfortable.

It is important to keep in mind that characteristics are not necessarily essential features. Characteristics serve to help us identify what sorts of things fit together within a category; they highlight what the philosopher Ludwig Wittgenstein referred to as a "family resemblance." Thus, identifying several characteristics might help us determine whether a particular place is an example of a third place, but the absence of one or more of those characteristics does not mean a particular place does not fit into the category. A set of characteristics, in other words, does not function as a checklist. This is important to keep in mind when considering whether venues that lack some of Oldenburg's characteristics—an online discussion forum or a neighbor's deck, for example—might serve as a third place.

One can usually tell whether a location qualifies as a "third place" as soon as one steps inside. Even two places that have very similar descriptions and serve similar functions may have a very different feel to them. Let me give an example.

Over the last few months, my wife and I have been touring microbreweries in our home state. Our most recent stop was Valkyrie Brewing Company in Dallas, Wisconsin. Established in 1994, the brewery is located in an old creamery building in the middle of town. A small tavern in the front made up of half a dozen tables with a bar in the corner greets the visitor at the brewery's entrance. As we walked through the door, the first thing we saw was a group of about ten people loosely gathered around a little table. You could see immediately how the group came to be. Most likely someone had come in early, sitting down at a table in the middle of the room. A little later someone else came in and joined them, then others arrived, pulling up nearby chairs. Even though everybody was gathered in a loosely formed circle around the table, there were several different conversations going on. They were telling stories and laughing, sharing a joke they had just heard, talking about the neighbor's boat that sank overnight, bragging about the size of their tomatoes. They were the regulars, and as I made my way up to the bar to order a beer, a man broke away from the group to join me, sharing his opinions on the various brews. Through the course of the evening, one or two people would leave and others would come in, drawn to the center of the room like metal filings to a magnet. The atmosphere was easygoing, relaxed, and lighthearted.

At the end of the evening, we paid our tab and said goodbye to those still gathered there. Heading out the door, we noticed two people we thought had left earlier in the evening. They were on the landing, one of them holding a broken piece of railing, deep in deliberation about how to repair it. It was not their building, yet they obviously regarded Valkyrie Brewing Company as "their" place, a "home away from home."

A few weeks later we visited Hillsboro Brewing Company, which is also located in a former creamery in a small town in rural Wisconsin, but that is where the similarity ends. When we walked through the door, we were greeted and ushered to a table, handed a menu, and told a server would be with us shortly. A Saturday afternoon in early summer, the place was packed; music was booming from a wedding reception on the upper floor. Children were running around exploring the various games placed throughout the building, and a row of television sets behind the expansive bar were showing baseball and golf. The service, the food, and the beer were all top-notch. It is a place we will almost certainly visit again, probably along with some friends. That's the kind of place it is. It is a destination, not a hangout. It is where you want to bring some friends, but it's not the sort of place where you can count on seeing old friends or would expect to make new friends. It is a thriving business and a fun place to go, yet many of the characteristics that make it successful also work against it functioning as a third place.

The contrast between Valkyrie Brewing Company and Hillsboro Brewing Company reveals something important about the challenges facing those who would like to create a third place. They tend to be small venues with relatively inexpensive offerings and a correspondingly limited capacity for economic return. That is not to say they are unprofitable, but they are generally not optimized solely for financial returns. The places are optimized for social interaction. Sometimes, these two aims can work together, but more often than not the pressure to make a place profitable works at odds with suitability for easygoing conversation and chance encounters.

There are exceptions, of course. My friend Curt is in his eighties and on a fixed income. He lives in a suburb of a small city. He and his retired friends meet every morning at a nearby McDonald's for coffee. If they had an inexpensive neighborhood café or coffee shop, they would probably meet there, but McDonald's is affordable and convenient, and they can sit and talk for a couple of hours without being asked to leave. In the absence of other options, McDonald's has become a third place across the country for many retired folks like Curt.

Several of the characteristics Oldenburg talks about—like accessibility, ordinariness, and the presence of regulars—means that third places tend to be located in neighborhoods, often in walking distance of the majority of people who go there. The owners or managers of such places also tend to care about people, and they intentionally create conditions in which conversations flourish and friendships are formed. It also happens to be the case that many such places are old. They are either family businesses, passed down for generations, or located in older buildings unsuited for a large-scale commercial enterprise.

Jenny's story illustrates the challenges of maintaining a third place that is also profitable. When she was hired as manager of a coffee shop that was struggling to keep the doors open, the first thing she did was try to soften the atmosphere. She brought in some old, comfortable sofas and offered free Wi-Fi service. One of the servers enjoyed making soup, so she added a different homemade soup to the menu each day. She worked with her staff to ensure every customer felt welcome and "at home." Gradually, business picked up. Before long there were several "regulars," people who showed up every day. Some spent long periods of time there and others just stopped in to pick up a coffee. But when new owners bought the business, they looked at the low customer turnover rate and calculated that there was more profit to be made. They told Jenny to remove the sofas and replace them with straight back chairs, thus discouraging customers from sitting too long. They also wanted her to turn up the music, making it more difficult for long conversations. They wanted the menu simplified, with the same offerings every day; that meant no more homemade soup. The changes were successful in driving away the few regulars who tended to stay way too long, but that did not mean the coffee shop enjoyed more customer turnover. Instead, they just had fewer customers. Within a year, the coffee shop closed.

The impediments to creating third places come not just from the challenge of making such an operation financially feasible, it also comes from the difficulty of getting a suitable design approved by local authorities.

James Howard Kunstler notes that "it is literally against the law almost everywhere in the United States to build the kind of places that Americans themselves consider authentic and traditional. It's against the law to build places that human beings can feel good in, or afford to live in. It's against the law to build places that are worth caring about."[4] He is commenting on the fact that zoning laws, which became ubiquitous in the years after World War II, completely changed the constructed landscape in which we live today. Those laws ruled out commercial businesses in residential neighborhoods, so no more corner groceries, delicatessens, cafés, or taverns. They mandated parking lots and setbacks from the street, so no more easy access for pedestrians. They specified the design, materials, and construction methods of many of the businesses we frequent, so every place looks the same. Today we have two types of buildings that stand out as distinctive: legacy buildings (constructed before World War II) or very expensive new buildings designed by architects to have some peculiar character or charm. The latter are generally too costly to function as third places. It is hard to get a return on a high-dollar investment if one of the building's chief purposes is to facilitate conversation.

But there are other challenges even greater than zoning laws or the cost of new buildings. Third places are competing with technologies that allow people to get the goods, services, and information they require with minimal social interaction.

Kathy and Dave own a small-town bowling alley and bar in northern Wisconsin. About fifteen years ago, they began noticing a gradual but significant drop in their business during the holidays. For as long as they could remember, people coming back home for the holidays would stop in at the bar to find out who was around and see old friends. But in recent years, people just weren't coming in anymore.

What accounted for the change? Kathy suspected it was social media. Folks were using Facebook or Instagram to find out what everyone was up to; they didn't need to stop in at the bar. So, Dave came up with an idea. Why not use social media to their advantage? They identified the followers of their Facebook page who had the most "friends" and offered them $100 certificates to the bowling alley. All they had to do was host an event with a group of ten or more people. The result? A big goose egg. Nada. Nobody used the certificates.

Dave explained it to me this way. The people to whom they gave certificates had a lot of friends on Facebook, but they didn't necessarily have deep connections. Some of them liked the idea of hosting a bowling party and tried to make it happen, but they couldn't get a group of people to show up.

When I ask my students to write about their own third place, it turns out most have difficulty completing the assignment. Most know exactly what it is and can identify places that meet Oldenburg's criteria. They can write about a third place they have visited, where they have seen others gather and talk and joke, but they do not regularly visit a place like that themselves. And they nearly always feel that fact reflects a deficit in their own lives. They are not alone. Few Americans today have a third place to call their own, yet most desire to have one. It is time to reverse the trend by working purposefully toward more socially connected communities. That work begins with understanding the role that third places play in bringing people together.

One might suppose that cities could build social gathering spaces by dedicating more resources to public projects, but, except for public parks, the places where people gather are overwhelmingly private. In 2021, the American Community Life Survey found that most Americans (about 70 percent) live close to neighborhood amenities of some kind, such as public parks, community centers, libraries, gyms, coffee shops, or taverns, but the places they tend to visit regularly are overwhelmingly commercial locations such as coffee shops, cafés, bars, and restaurants. About a quarter of Americans regularly go to a public park or community garden, while only 3 percent regularly go to libraries or community centers. That means we should be paying more attention to policies that encourage private development of the sorts of places where people like to hang out.

The benefits are enormous. People who have a regular third place greatly expand their circle of friends; they laugh more often; they are more engaged in their community; they are happier; they live longer. But third places do more than just make individuals more satisfied with their lives—they also benefit entire communities. As we shall see, third places serve as gateways so people new to the area can get to know their neighbors; they function as incubators for new ideas; they serve as safety nets for people in crisis; they build social trust; they decrease political polarization.

Cities that do not encourage the development of third places or which sit idly by while the older places where people once gathered gradually close, end up paying the price. A team of researchers at the University of Michigan and Princeton University have come up with what they call the Index of Deep Disadvantage. Writing about the conditions in central Appalachia, they learned about the devastating effects of drug use in the region, but they also discovered underlying causes that rarely get mentioned. Talking to residents of Manchester, in Clay County, Kentucky, they heard about the loss of places like the local movie theater, several bars and cafés, beauty salons, and a park that was destroyed for the sake of a highway project. When asked about the rise of opioid use in the county, people living there bemoaned the fact that there is now "nothing to do but drugs."

The decline of social interaction across the United States was convincingly documented in Robert Putnam's classic book *Bowling Alone: The Collapse and Revival of American Community*. Putnam's work was published in 2000, and he attributed the decline to several factors that significantly changed society in the 1950s, '60s, and '70s—things like automobiles, suburban sprawl, and television. In subsequent decades, innovations in computers had an even greater impact, and social interaction continued to decline at an even faster pace. Smartphones and social media are simply the latest developments in a trend of technological advances that collectively serve to make us less dependent on one another for our daily needs.

Think of how companies like Netflix, Hulu, and Sling changed home entertainment. They provided more choices by expanding the number of programs available to watch, and they made our lives easier by removing the inconvenience of trips to the local video store. But they also removed numerous small opportunities for social interaction by making it more desirable to stay at home by ourselves, sitting alone by the cool blue hearth.

Amazon did the same thing with home delivery. The freedom of shopping at home comes at a cost, and not just the cost of shipping or the economic loss of local retail stores. It comes at the cost of meeting one's neighbors—saying hello to an old acquaintance in the shoe aisle, catching up on the news of the summer, the birth of a granddaughter, the latest antics of Uncle Bob.

Online ordering from restaurants, along with food delivery services like Uber Eats and DoorDash, make even the most basic of human activities—preparing, serving, and eating food—a process that can be done without ever talking to another human being. The intention is to make the consumer experience more "friendly," which is the new corporate speak for convenience. The result greatly reduces opportunities for human interaction. That does not necessarily make our communities unfriendly, but it tends to make our experiences out in public nonfriendly— more impersonal, sterile, and cold. All of this is part of an effort by businesses to create a "frictionless" experience for consumers. That is a corporate trend sure to be enhanced in the coming years by improvements in robotics and AI. Yet, it is worth keeping in mind that friction is what generates warmth.

Robust social interaction is essential for a healthy society. When the French political philosopher Alexis de Tocqueville visited America in 1831, he remarked on the inclination of people to form together in voluntary associations: "In the United States, as soon as several inhabitants have taken an opinion or an idea they wish to promote in society, they seek each other out and unite together once they have made contact. From that moment, they are no longer isolated but have become a power seen from afar whose activities serve as an example and whose words are heeded."[5]

We can think of social capital as a reservoir of trust generated whenever citizens gather in some sort of shared enterprise, creating collaborative networks that advance the common good. Houses of worship, service clubs, gyms, libraries, book clubs, rod and gun clubs, neighborhood taverns, festivals, sporting leagues—all contribute to the health of society by fostering social capital. They provide opportunities for citizens to interact on a regular basis and in meaningful ways, becoming gradually more familiar with one another. The resulting trust, based on a shared commitment to making decisions through public deliberation, is what allows a democracy to flourish.

But social capital is a threatened resource. Americans are retreating from public life and becoming increasingly private. The term "idiot" comes from an ancient Greek term meaning "private person." The Greeks, who devised the democratic form of government, thought failure to participate in some form of public life could only come from inability, not free choice. But we are increasingly choosing to withdraw from public participation, and we are building cities and towns that make it more difficult to get involved.

Communities with a high degree of social capital have people who are more likely to participate, share ideas, and work toward the common good than those in communities with low social capital. People in such communities also report that they trust one another and the institutions upon which they depend.

Why is this important? Think of the amount of money local, state, and federal governments spend on fixing problems like crime, domestic violence, obesity, drug abuse, and homelessness. Yet, we know from years of extensive research into social capital that (a) communities with a high degree of social capital also have much better outcomes on virtually every measure: education, health, children's welfare, socioeconomic mobility, and safety; and (b) communities with many third places have greater social capital. So, you would think it would be a no-brainer for elected officials to make it a priority to build social capital by enacting policies that promote third places. But, with a few exceptions, that is not what happens. Instead, we get more dollars poured into development that separates housing from workplaces and builds more transportation to take people from one area to another. And that is because, despite the attention it has received in recent years, social capital is still largely misunderstood and underappreciated.

The reasons for that are complex. First, it is hard to see the causal connection between something like trust, which is difficult to define and measure, and outcomes like health or safety, which can be defined and measured with comparative ease. Second, trust does not work by replacing investments in social outcomes; instead, it works by enhancing those investments. Communities with high levels of trust are composed of people who enjoy working together and know how to do it. Communities with low levels of trust have people who undermine one another or who refuse to collaborate because they are pursuing their own interests. They believe defeating their opponents' aims is more important than achieving shared goals. In a democratic society, lasting good can only be produced by consensus. When a political faction uses its power to leverage policies that do not have popular support, the immediate results are generally short-lived. The long-term results are public cynicism and political upheaval.

Several years ago, I was asked to serve on a local council tasked with reducing the jail population. The jail was over capacity and the county board did not want to approve an addition to a structure that had just been completed a few years before. The council was made up of some citizen representatives, a couple of county board members, and several criminal justice professionals, including judges, attorneys, and law enforcement officers. Even though nobody was formally affiliated with a political party, those with conservative leanings would sit on one side of the table and those with liberal leanings on the other. When anybody from one side proposed a strategy, the other side would oppose it. We met at 7:00 a.m. every two weeks for six months and accomplished nothing at all.

Then somebody had the brilliant idea of bringing coffee and donuts to the meeting. Instead of everybody walking straight over to their usual seat at the table, folks would gather around the donuts and end up talking to whoever happened to be standing next to them. They would have conversations about how their children or grandchildren were doing in school, where they had traveled over the summer, or how their gardens were growing. Picking up their refreshments, they would wander over to a couple of open seats and continue their conversation.

After a few weeks I noticed during the meeting that right- and left-leaning council members were scattered randomly around the table, and because it was no longer quite as evident whether proposals were coming from the "right" side or the "wrong" side, they were listening to one another a little bit more. Over the following months we began to make slow but steady progress, reducing the jail population by improving the intake process, reducing courthouse delays, and eliminating ineffective programs. Neither side won the debate; instead, we got rid of the sides and started to focus on fixing the problem.

Whenever we get into oppositional attitudes we tend to exaggerate policy differences in order to define ourselves and our opponents. We stop looking at evidence and focus instead on defending our position, which ends up driving people to support extreme solutions that are unlikely to work. We assume that anyone who supports a different policy disagrees with our goals.

The truth is, most people share similar goals. We all want prosperity, health, and security, and we know less than we think about how to obtain them. We need to listen to one another, carefully evaluating what may or may not work, and then give different policies a try, seeing whether they turn out the way we expect. Policies are just tools, and tools are only as effective as the people who use them.

A great example illustrating the importance of trust within communities is a study conducted by Anthony Bryk and Barbara Schneider. Over a period of three years, they looked at efforts directed toward educational reform in twelve Chicago elementary schools. By focusing on the relationships among teachers, students, parents, and administrators, they found that schools with high levels of trust among all their constituents were much more willing to work together to experiment with new practices and, as a result, had significant improvements in student learning. The schools with low levels of trust saw no gains. They concluded that trust is more important than most of the policies that typically occupy the attention of would-be educational reformers.

Building consensus requires trust, which is produced by social capital. No social capital, no trust. No trust, no consensus. No consensus, no political stability. No political stability, no lasting good.

Social capital comes in two forms: bonding capital and bridging capital. Bonding capital forms when friends and acquaintances get together to share mutual interests. An example would be a regular gathering of friends at a coffee shop or a book club. Such gatherings tend to strengthen existing social ties by deepening friendships. Bridging capital is when people from diverse backgrounds and identities come together for a common purpose. Organizations like Habitat for Humanity and the Red Cross rely upon bridging capital to achieve their ends. A society's ability to create and sustain bridging capital is the primary indicator of health and resiliency, yet bonding capital is necessary for bridging capital to grow. And third places are incubators for bonding capital. To understand why, consider the story of Rotary Lights.

When Pat Stephens heard about a large holiday light display from a friend, he thought it would be an interesting project for his local Rotary Club. The friend had just returned from Oklahoma, where he had visited his daughter's college and witnessed the lights. Could they do something similar in La Crosse, Wisconsin? Pat contacted the people who organized the Magnificent Mile Lights Festival in Chicago to find out where they purchased their lights; they directed him to a company in Rockford, Illinois. Bringing other area Rotary Clubs together to raise funds, they put in an order for 250,000 lights.

Negotiations with the city resulted in approval to locate the display in Riverside Park, near the downtown shopping area. A local utility company donated space in a warehouse to store their equipment: large spools of lights, ladders, extension cords, signs, and multiple structures that had to be assembled and disassembled. So far things were going well, but the project really took off after a chance conversation at a coffee shop one morning. Pat and his friends were discussing the light display, wondering whether it could serve some greater purpose. Someone suggested asking attendees to donate a food item. That sounded like a good idea, so they added it to the plan. In 1995, the first year of Rotary Lights, they collected 13,500 food items, which they gave to the Salvation Army.

Twenty-nine years later, the project has grown beyond the imagination of everyone involved with the initial project. Today there are four million lights displayed from Thanksgiving to New Year's Eve. They collect more than 300,000 food items annually, which are distributed to fourteen area food pantries, along with checks ranging from $1,000 to $5,000. In 2022, they purchased a $22,000 walk-in cooler for the YMCA and large refrigerators for the Boys and Girls Club and Big Brothers, Big Sisters. In addition, they contributed $32,000 to a capital campaign for Wafer, the largest food pantry in the region. To date, Pat and his team have helped sixteen other communities establish their own holiday light display. In return for their assistance, they only ask that the project be a nonprofit with the mission of feeding the hungry.

It takes three thousand volunteers every winter to make Rotary Lights happen, but they would never come together if a greater purpose had not been generated by a few people tossing out ideas over a cup of coffee. It is an example of how bonding capital underlies bridging capital. It is often a conversation among friends (bonding) that generates new ideas and provides the initial impetus for a project, but it takes a larger number of people with a shared purpose but weaker social ties (bridging) to bring the project to fruition and maintain it. In thriving communities, it is generally unclear just where bonding capital ends and bridging capital begins, because people may belong to multiple friendship groups and be involved in several larger associations as well. They are regularly moving in and out of circles with stronger and weaker ties. Moreover, many service organizations (like Rotary, Kiwanis, and Lions), and many houses of worship as well, utilize both bonding and bridging capital, bringing people together in small groups to get to know and like one another well and then organizing fundraising projects or volunteer activities that rely on the collaboration of larger numbers of people with weaker ties. The key thing to keep in mind is that bridging capital flourishes only where bonding capital is already present. It is the strong ties of friendship that create conditions in which people are likely to have enough trust to invest themselves in collaboration with strangers. It is also in friendship groups that people are likely to learn more about opportunities for wider involvement and be invited to participate.

If we look at the record of great collaborative achievements in history, we will frequently come across mentions of a gathering of friends at some third place that turns out to be an essential factor in the achievement's story. An example is Aldo Leopold's account of the Coon Valley Erosion Project in 1934.

> Not all the sights of Coon Valley are to be seen by day. No less distinctive is the nightly "bull session" of the technical staff. One may hear a forester expounding to an engineer the basic theory of how organic matter in the soil decreases the per cent of run-off; an economist holds forth on tax rebates as a means to get farmers to install their own erosion control. Underneath the facetious conversation one detects a vein of thought—an attitude toward the common enterprise—which is strangely reminiscent of the early days of the Forest Service. Then, too, a staff of technicians,

all under thirty, was faced by a common task so
large and so long as to stir the imagination of
all but dullards. I suspect that the Soil Erosion
Service, perhaps unwittingly, has recreated a
spiritual entity which many older conservation-
ists have thought long since dead.[6]

Who could have imagined that the key to success
of the nation's first large-scale watershed restoration
would not be a detailed plan worked out around
the conference table of Washington bureaucrats but
rather nightly conversations around a campfire? Far
from home and no doubt exhausted from a hard
day's work, the young men of the Soil Erosion Service found a place to socialize. They found friendship.
They found belonging. They found purpose. In the
most unlikely of circumstances, they found a third
place on a hillside in rural Wisconsin. Bonding and
bridging. Without places to cultivate friendship, civilization cannot maintain itself.

CHAPTER THREE

# Work and Leisure

*This is the main question, with what activity should one's leisure be filled.*

Aristotle, *Politics*

"**S**ometimes I just feel like giving up." These words were uttered by a person I've always admired for his energy and enthusiasm, his passion for worthy causes, and his ability to encourage others to achieve more than they thought possible. Yet I knew just how he felt: tired, underappreciated, and wondering whether the extra effort really made any difference. He was experiencing burnout, which afflicts nearly everyone at some point in their life.

At the time of our conversation, I was going through a period of burnout as well. The job I had loved wasn't interesting anymore. I would wake up in the morning thinking about a vacation still six months away. I would leave the house tired and return in the evening feeling the same way.

I wondered about a colleague who seemed to have inexhaustible energy and enthusiasm. She was older than I was, well past the age when most people retire, yet she was still working and volunteering and enjoying every minute of life. When asked how she managed to stay so productive, she just laughed: "If you are going to burn the candle at both ends, you just have to get more wax." Some people seem to have an inexhaustible supply of wax, but they are the exceptional few, and there are fewer every year. Workplace statistics indicate we are a nation filled with people running out of wax.

Herbert Freudenberger coined the term "burnout" forty years ago. He described it as a "state of mental and physical exhaustion caused by one's professional life." Burnout rates have been increasing steadily during the past two decades. The American Psychological Association, in its annual Work and Well-being Survey, found in 2021 that 79 percent of employees reported work-related stress in the prior month. A 2017 survey by the American Federation of Teachers found that 61 percent reported high levels of stress. A Mayo Clinic study in 2017 revealed burnout among 55 percent of physicians. You can go down the list of occupations. From nurses to social workers to custodians to athletes, work-related stress is at an all-time high.

For years, we have been told that the cure for burnout is that elusive state termed "work-life balance." Achieving the balance, we are told, is a matter of getting away: spending more time on "life" and less time on "work." For some who experience burnout, that may be true. They might be working long hours at a job that requires extreme physical, mental, or emotional exertion. They just need some time to recover, to restore their bodies and their minds. For most people, however, the cause of burnout is not so evident, nor is the remedy. They are afflicted by a deepening listlessness, a lethargy that infects every aspect of their lives. For them, taking time away does not restore their energy so they can return to work revitalized. They turn to vacation, not as a time for relaxation and renewal but as an opportunity for escape.

That is the state I was in. I was thinking more and more about getting away—away from people, away from commitments and deadlines, away from everything that up until that point defined my professional life. But getting away did not help for long. Everything I tried just seemed to deepen my lethargy.

The very phrase "work-life balance" is misleading. It suggests a teeter-totter, with work on one end and life on the other. The problem is, when you have a bad day at work, it carries over to your home, and when things are not going well at home, you bring those concerns with you into the workplace. So, the key is not so much where one spends one's time but rather how one spends it, and I was evidently spending my time on the wrong things.

I decided to take an inventory of my activities. I drew three overlapping circles on a blank sheet of paper. I labeled each circle as a different area of life: professional, personal, and social. I thought about the various activities I did throughout the week and wrote each one down in its appropriate circle. Some activities fell into more than one area; they were placed in the overlapping sections. I didn't worry too much about where the activities belonged; I was more worried about their effect on my overall energy. Next to the activities that increased my energy I placed a "+" sign. Those that depleted my energy got a "-" sign. The result was a picture of my energy levels.

What I discovered surprised me. In all three areas of my life—at work, at home, and in social settings—I was spending most of my time on energy-draining activities. Looking at some of the things that gave me energy, I found that I was doing much less than in previous years—less teaching, less writing, less time outdoors, less time socializing with people outside of work. No wonder I was feeling lethargic. I needed to make a change.

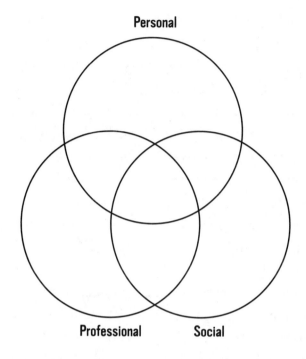

The challenge was to balance the time I spent on pluses and minuses. I decided to strictly limit the time I spent each day reading and responding to emails. I gave up some committee assignments and budgeted the amount of attention I gave to administrative duties. Most significantly, I realized that the social area of my life was filled with volunteer work that involved lots of meetings, paperwork, and screen time—the same things I found so energy-draining in my professional life. I promptly resigned from a committee at my church and from a board that I had been serving on for several years. I looked for volunteer activities that would allow me to interact with people directly rather than work behind the scenes on policies and budgets. At work, I offered to teach an extra class each semester, began exercising more regularly, and committed to writing a regular newspaper column. Finally, I asked a few friends if they would like to get together every week for an early breakfast. We all agreed to put the weekly breakfast meeting on our schedules, knowing that if we did not, the time would get used up by other more urgent but less important activities. Within a few weeks I noticed that I was working harder, getting more done, and feeling much happier—at home, at work, and in the community. I discovered that the attempt at "balance" was the wrong way to think about the cause of my lethargy. It wasn't a matter of having less work and more life; it was a matter of working and living differently, more intentionally. And the key to that was recognizing the need for more meaningful social connections, the kind one finds in third places.

It may seem paradoxical, but the person who is experiencing burnout is generally not suffering from too much work, but from the wrong kind of work, or the wrong kinds of leisure activities, or both. None of us gets to eliminate from our lives all the things that drain energy. Much of my day is still filled with answering emails, reading and writing reports, and sitting through committee meetings. The key is not simply working less, but finding activities—at work, at home, in the community—that give one enough energy to get through the more tedious but necessary tasks that make up the bulk of each day.

What kinds of activities give a person energy? The particulars differ considerably from one person to another, but there are some general characteristics. First, they tend to be meaningful; that is, they contribute to some worthwhile goal. Second, they are creative, either making or transforming something into a form that is new and interesting. Third, and most important, they are relational, broadening and deepening one's connection to others.

Many people choose to do activities during their leisure time that turn out to be energy draining rather than restorative. Watching television, for example, may be easy and enjoyable, but the longer one spends doing it, the less energy one feels afterward. It is significant that the average American spends close to three hours per day watching television. It is something that is easy to do, but it is not meaningful, creative, or relational.

When Thoreau famously observed that "the mass of men lead lives of quiet desperation," he was talking about something very similar to what we mean by "burnout" today. It is what medieval theologians called *acedia*, a listlessness of spirit. The Hebrews introduced the sabbath as an antidote to burnout. The seventh day was not simply a break from work but also a time for renewal, a place from which to gain perspective, to pray, to study, to reflect on the meaning of life in community with others.

The ancient Greeks spoke of *schola*, from which we get the term "school," but which is most precisely translated as "leisure." Whereas we tend to think the purpose of schools and universities is preparing young people for work, the Greeks thought of work as the price one pays to have leisure. Work is what one must do to survive; leisure is what one chooses to do—it is what provides us with a perspective from which to understand the purpose of life. As Josef Pieper observes, "Leisure is a form of that stillness that is the necessary preparation for accepting reality; only the person who is still can hear, and whoever is not still, cannot hear."[7]

Americans put a great deal of energy into improving the workplace. We have seminars on employee engagement, policies to prevent bullying and harassment, programs to encourage fitness, and specialists in workplace ergonomics. But for all our attention to workplace improvement, we do a lousy job of managing our leisure time. That's partly due to language. Nearly all our words to denote leisure are negative, marking off a time in our lives that is left over from work. The "weekend" denotes the days left over after the "work week." "Time off" is time we take not to work; "sick days" are for when we cannot work. The word "vacation" comes from the Latin word *vacare*, "to be unoccupied." "Retirement" comes from the French word "to withdraw," implying a time of life when one stops being active.

If one's time away from work is not used wisely, then our leisure time ends up being occupied by meaningless diversions, ways of spending useless time rather than filling up our lives with something worthwhile. Activity follows activity until we find ourselves doing "one damn thing after another," a condition that contributes to burnout instead of preventing it. If leisure is our best opportunity for finding fulfillment, and yet all our words for times of leisure imply negation, is it any wonder that so many people feel afflicted by emptiness?

In his autobiography, Benjamin Franklin included "industry" among his key virtues. (You might recall Franklin as the author of popular sayings like "Early to bed, early to rise, makes a man healthy, wealthy, and wise.") Today when people think of industriousness, they think about productivity and employment statistics, but Franklin thought of it more broadly. He characterized it this way: "lose no time; be always employed in something useful; cut off all unnecessary actions." "Industry" is another word for what today we call "effort." Franklin was a businessman, a politician, and a scholar, and the virtue of industry applied to all three areas of his life. Familiar with ancient Greek literature, Franklin regarded politics and education as leisure activities, something one did when one was not working. But they required dedication and attention, so industry applied to them as well.

During the past two hundred years much has changed, especially in the most developed parts of the world, and that change is mostly due to what came to be called "industrialization," a corruption of the original meaning of "industry." With automation came an increase in productivity, but a decrease in meaningful work. As workplaces came to be dominated by machines, the role of human beings in the workplace changed, often assuming roles in large, complex systems in which machines dictated the pace and the content of the work. As we saw in chapter one, this led to a massive increase in prosperity all over the world, but it also led to more dissatisfaction in our lives.

Industrialization meant that many people did not have to master a craft to participate in economic life, they just had to learn a series of tasks. In the modern economy, workers participate in a system, and their worth is evaluated entirely on productivity. Systems tend by nature toward the impersonal and noncreative. By contrast, mastering a craft means being initiated into a way of life. It takes a long time, usually many years, and those years are spent in relationship with others who are either teaching the craft or learning it also, and one's worth is measured not just by what one produces but also by how one contributes to the community. When Studs Terkel observed in his book *Working* that "work is about a search for daily meaning as well as daily bread, for recognition as well as cash, for astonishment rather than torpor; in short, for a sort of life rather than a Monday through Friday sort of dying,"[8] he was expressing sorrow for the changing American workplace, the fact that so many people had jobs in which they could take no pride. Efficiency had replaced effort as the measure of worth in the workplace, and you cannot take pride in the efficiency of the system if you simply perform a set of tasks to keep the system running, especially if those tasks could be done by anyone with a bit of training.

One of the things that has happened to our cities is that we have built them on the model of the factory, with every component serving to make the whole more productive. That productivity is measured largely by growth. But cities are not just economic engines, and the economy is not the only measure of well-being for humans living together. We need to base our cities on an understanding of what it means to live a good human life—what Aristotle called *eudaimonia*, or "flourishing." This means our cities should be places where we have multiple opportunities for meaningful social interaction so that children may grow up to have complete, fully human lives. In other words, our cities must not only be places for work but places for leisure as well.

I can remember a time and a place when industrialization had not yet taken over many of the small towns and rural areas, when social life and work life were more integrated. Growing up in a small Midwestern town in the 1960s and '70s meant having multiple daily opportunities for talking to a variety of people, and the workplace was where much of that talk occurred.

My father had a small store on Main Street where he sold paint, glass, wallpaper, and antique furniture. My grandfather, Emmett, had a real estate office located inside the store, just large enough for his desk and a couple of chairs for customers. Most mornings Emmett would head across the street to play pinochle for an hour or so with his buddies in the lobby of the old theater. All day long people would stop by, help themselves to a cup of coffee from the pot near the counter, and catch up on the day's gossip. Sometime after lunch, Leonard, whose family owned the little grocery store next door, would come over to play a couple of hands of cribbage with Emmett. At the end of the day, my father would hang a "closed" sign on the front door, turn out the lights, and head to the workshop at the back of the store. Ray, who lived just across the alley, would wander in through the back door, usually joined by one or two others who happened to be in town. They would sit on stools in the workshop drinking cheap beer and telling stories until it was time to go home.

In that place and time, the workplace was not reserved solely for work, and neither was the home. My grandmother, Mae, always had a pot of coffee on the stove and some kind of dessert prepared in case guests stopped by. It wasn't unusual for friends to show up unannounced and spend two or three hours visiting, especially on the weekends. Most people we knew had a part of the house reserved for social functions—the living room, the dining room, the front porch. Even those who did not have rooms ready to receive guests would go out of their way to make them comfortable when they arrived. It was a widely shared cultural norm.

The word "visit" is one of those rare words that has changed very little from its origins; it still retains its Latin meaning of "to go see." To visit a person or a place is to go and see for oneself, to spend time in the presence of another, but the practice has declined in recent years. As our nation has prospered, we have become more self-reliant, using cell phones and computers to mediate our interactions with one another. Gone are the days when a spontaneous visit was a commonplace way to spend a Sunday afternoon.

Because social life in the community was so fully integrated with work and home, the people in my town did not require third places to get to know one another. There were third places, to be sure, like Sue's Café, Dave's Bakery, the United Methodist Church basement, and the municipal tavern. But such places merely expanded the opportunities for a robust social life that was already present in the community. Few people today live in communities where the different aspects of our lives can be so richly integrated. The workplace is where we work. The home is where we conduct our personal lives. We need dedicated places to form and nurture social relationships, or else we go without.

I do not mean to idealize the small-town life of a half century ago. Some problems come with having work life, personal life, and social life so closely connected. It can be confining, especially if one does not fit in with the expectations of others. Privacy can be hard to come by. Small-town gossip can be noxious. Nor did everyone participate. Some just chose to opt out: they did not take time to visit other people, they did not receive guests in their homes; when they went downtown, they just did their business and left. But the point is this: for those who wanted social connection, it was easy.

There are still people who manage to make a living on the edges of the mainstream corporate world, but it is getting harder to live entirely outside an economic system based on production. Small stores in rural communities continue to close, pushed out of business by large box stores and internet sales. And even if individuals here and there manage to resist the push to participate in an economy governed by the laws of productivity and efficiency, the communities around them have already changed. It is hard to maintain social connections on an island.

In Gallup's annual survey, they regularly find that about 30 percent of American workers are "engaged" in their work, and, of those, only 10 percent are "actively engaged." That means 70 percent are either "not engaged" or "actively disengaged." The numbers are surprisingly consistent across various occupations. Doctors, nurses, teachers, construction workers, office workers, salesclerks, and truck drivers all fall between 25 and 35 percent engagement.

No occupation even comes close to having half of its members engaged in their work.

Part of the explanation comes from the observation that what matters most to people is not just the type of work they are doing but the people with whom they are doing it. According to Gallup, "Managers account for at least 70% of the variance in employee engagement scores across business units."[9] In other words, even in a company with overall low engagement levels, a single manager can make work interesting and meaningful for the people he or she supervises. On the other hand, a single manager can make life miserable in a company that is for most others a great place to be. What do good managers do to help their people stay engaged? It is simple. They treat people like people and not like things.

The best companies, those with the highest performance and worker satisfaction ratings, do not sacrifice humanity for the sake of profits. An example is Cisco Systems, an information technology company based in California. For three straight years, they have topped *Fortune* magazine's list of the one hundred best companies to work for, with 98 percent of their employees saying it is a great place to work. They find ways to respect their employees by sincerely soliciting and responding to feedback, focusing on the purpose of their work, and ensuring that everyone's contribution is valued. They encourage their employees to get to know one another socially, and they emphasize the importance of having managers who demonstrate empathy and support. But there are limits to what even the best companies can do because they function within a larger cultural context that has fully adopted the language and the norms of "systems thinking."

That larger cultural context is significant because the changing nature of the workplace is only one side of the industrialization coin; the other side is the changing nature of our leisure activities. Technological progress has profoundly changed the size and arrangement of our public spaces. If you think about the way our physical spaces affect our relations to one another, you will begin to understand two things: first, why our leisure activities over the past century have changed from mostly active (playing games together) to mostly passive (being entertained); second, why our entertainments, as well as our politics, have become increasingly dark.

Prior to the mid-twentieth century, most social interaction took place in small circles in which everyone participated in some form of creative activity: playing cards, telling stories, singing, dancing. The places where people gathered for such activities were dance halls, church basements, ice rinks, town halls, public squares—spaces no larger than the human voice could carry without amplification and where everybody's face could be seen from anywhere in the venue. But when movie projectors, screens, and sound systems came along, places like movie theaters, civic centers, and sporting arenas proliferated, which do not require participation but only showing up to watch.

Once entertainment became largely passive, it only took more technological innovation to provide the same thing in homes, just on a smaller scale. Radios and television meant that we could listen to the same entertainers and see the same programs in the privacy of our homes. The important point is this: as entertainment changed, so did people's orientation to one another—from face-to-face to side-by-side and, finally, to alone in the dark.

Anybody who has ever attended a meeting or sat in a classroom with chairs lined up in rows has experienced the difference between that and being in a room in which everybody is seated around a table. When people are face-to-face, they tend to pay attention to one another. When they are seated side-by-side, they tend to interact much less. They might carry on a conversation with the person sitting right next to them, but the group as a whole will not participate in the conversation. When people are on a Zoom call, they interact even less.

Sitting around a table or a campfire, as generations of our ancestors did, primes people for collaboration. Sitting in rows with everyone facing the same direction primes people either for compliance or defiance. Sitting alone in the dark primes people for conspiracy.

As our orientation to one another changed, so did our tastes in entertainment. Consider, for example, the current popularity of true crime programs. Fascination with crime, especially sensational, monstrous crime, is nothing new. In Great Britain in the nineteenth century, publishers of penny dreadfuls were selling more than a million copies a week. They featured violent exploits of characters like Sweeney Todd and Spring-Heeled Jack. In this country, many dime novels of the same era told lurid stories about outlaws like Billy the Kid and Jesse James.

The difference today is not so much in the nature of the storytelling as in the sheer volume of it. In the 1930s and '40s, Warner Brothers was making three or four highly popular gangster movies like *Public Enemy* and *Scarface* every year. Universal Studios was thrilling audiences with horror films like *Frankenstein* and *The Invisible Man* at about the same pace. A devoted fan of frightening entertainment could maybe watch a movie every month and then listen to radio programs like *The Shadow* or *The Whistler* a few times a week.

Today, the entertainment industry feeds us a steady diet of the horrific. True crime is especially popular, featured in podcasts, audiobooks, movies, documentaries, and TV series. In 2022, the miniseries *Monster: The Jeffrey Dahmer Story* set viewing records for Netflix. The most popular genre on podcasts is true crime, with shows like *Crime Junkie*, *My Favorite Murder*, *Serial*, *In the Dark*, and *Morbid* appearing regularly in top ten lists. Bingeing on programs that depict the worst of humanity is today not just possible, it is a way of life for many.

Well, some might say, what's wrong with that? After all, stories are just stories. Watching crime shows doesn't turn one into a criminal any more than watching monster movies turns one into a monster. That's true enough. But stories do affect us. They enter our imagination, and the more time we spend with certain kinds of stories the more they shape the way we see the world around us. They subtly influence whether we are more inclined to see a stranger as a potential threat or a potential friend. They can influence our decisions about where to live, what legislation to support, and which politicians to vote for. As Iris Murdoch observed, "We make pictures of ourselves and come to resemble the pictures."[10]

A friend who recently moved to a home in the country mentioned she was having trouble sleeping.

"I keep hearing strange noises," she said, "and I think somebody is trying to get into the house." When I talked to her a few weeks later, she was sleeping fine. "I just had to quit listening to those true crime podcasts," she laughed. "They were playing with my mind." That's it exactly. The stories we consume play with our minds, and if we aren't careful, they can make us lose our minds altogether.

In the *Republic*, a book in which Plato imagines the construction of an ideal society, he argues that storytellers should be banned. He does so not because there is anything wrong with stories as such, but because the stories that tend to appeal to us most are sensational ones depicting the worst behavior. Stories of murder, rape, and torture have an immediate, visceral appeal. Stories about goodness, on the other hand, seem boring by comparison. Who wants to see a movie about somebody helping their neighbor rake the leaves or baking a cake for a community fundraiser?

Yet, the quality of our lives depends on most people spending most of their time doing just such things—quietly going about the business of working hard, raising children, helping neighbors, and participating in the life of their community. Besides, it is simply not true that goodness is boring, it's just that the most interesting aspects of goodness are participative. They do not lend themselves to spectacle. It is not very exciting to watch corn grow, but the life of the farmer who plants, tends, and harvests crops can be richly rewarding.

In Mary Shelley's *Frankenstein*, Viktor Frankenstein observes, "If the study to which you apply yourself has a tendency to weaken your affections and to destroy your taste for those simple pleasures in which no alloy can possibly mix, then that study is certainly unlawful, that is to say, not befitting the human mind."[11] The more time we spend entertaining ourselves with fantastic diversions that turn us away from one another instead of nurturing our lives in creative and sociable occupation, the worse we become. And, as we saw in chapter one, that worsening can be measured; we are becoming more anxious, more depressed, and more distrustful with every passing decade.

We are seeing evidence of that worsening not only in our popular culture but in our politics as well. We carry on our political debates as if the only thing that matters is policy, and in the name of improving our nation through better policy, we excuse the worst lapses of moral character, sacrifice friendships, and destroy institutions. It is an approach to politics that gets everything backward. To get things right, we cannot simply complain about incivility or insist on placing more rules on people to force them to get along. In fact, Plato reminds us that a proliferation of laws is one of the signs of an unjust society. It means that citizens are unable to govern themselves and instead seek to regulate behavior through external means. What we need to do instead is change how we are oriented toward one another in our everyday lives, and that begins with thinking carefully about how our physical places serve to turn us together or turn us away from one another.

I will close this chapter with a final story illustrating the importance of physical places in changing our orientation toward one another, changes that have the power to greatly influence the culture of a household, a business, a community, or even a nation.

I teach at a small university that for most of its history had a building in the center of campus where the mail center was located. Just about everybody who worked on campus would find themselves heading over to the second floor of Murphy Center at least once a day to send and receive letters, pick up packages, or make copies. There was a wide section in the hallway lined with rows of brass post-office boxes. The area served as a place for "scuttlebutt" (an old-fashioned word for gossip, taken from the name for water fountains on naval ships, around which sailors would gather). Folks would go to pick up their mail, perhaps grabbing a cup of coffee from one of the nearby offices, and end up having a conversation with people from other parts of the university. You never knew who you would run into or what you would end up talking about, and I noticed that by the end of my first year, I knew just about everyone on the campus, even those who worked in buildings that I rarely had a reason to enter. But then something happened.

The university was making plans for a new building to be located on the corner of campus, and someone suggested it would be an ideal location for a new mailroom. The old mailroom in Murphy Center was severely outdated. The hallways were frequently congested, especially when students were going to and from classes, and its location on the second floor meant staff had to move boxes up and down an old, slow-moving elevator several times a day. The new building seemed ideal: the mailroom could be placed on the lower level of the building where it would not get in the way, there would be plenty of room for expansion as the university grew, and, most importantly, the building backed up to an alley where a loading dock could be built. Nobody thought to consider how moving the mailroom would change the campus culture.

Once the new building was completed, people changed their patterns of behavior. Because it was located next to the main parking lot, people tended to pick up their mail early in the mornings as they arrived or at the end of the day as they left. Those who worked in buildings on the other side of campus began sending somebody over to pick up mail for several people instead of everyone going themselves. The hallway was cold and sterile, usually empty, and nobody had an office nearby with a pot of coffee. I don't think most people noticed the cultural change on our campus right away, or if they did, they chalked it up to a change in policies or administration. But what I noticed was that every year after that more people were working on campus who I did not recognize, and the spirit of community and collaboration, which we had always taken for granted, became something we talked about trying to revive. After a few years, it was clear that everyone felt the change, even if it was hard to pinpoint a specific cause.

It seems to me that what has happened during my lifetime reflects a corruption of the ideas of both work and leisure. Workplace decisions are increasingly made with productivity as the only key metric, and leisure is thought of chiefly in terms of entertainment. As a result, the idea that both work and leisure should contribute to helping us live more fully human lives is lost. How we spend our leisure time is especially significant because it shapes our personal and collective character. Part of the task of reestablishing

a robust, integrated life that allows for human flourishing is recovering the idea of leisure as a time for
meaningful activity and the idea of work as allowing
us opportunities for contributing to the common
good. Both work and leisure should take us out of
the impersonality of systems thinking and orient us
toward instead of away from one another.

Third places are not the only location for this
positive notion of leisure, but they are places set aside,
especially for leisure. They serve as the scuttlebutts
of communities. They are where people meet one
another, exchange gossip, share ideas, and build trust.
They are the birthplaces of creativity and collaboration. They are where we go to get more wax.

CHAPTER FOUR
# Friendship

*True happiness is really only to be found
in sympathetic sharing.*

Johann Wolfgang Goethe,

Letter to Sarah von Grotthuss

My Facebook page says I have several hundred "friends." Most of them are acquaintances rather than friends, which is not to say I don't like them, respect them, or enjoy their company. It is just to say that my relationship with them, no matter how pleasant, is casual. We have a few things in common and interact now and then, whether virtually or in person, but we are not close.

The tendency to name all one's acquaintances "friends" is a symptom of the conceptual confusion that afflicts a culture careless with language. To point out this carelessness may seem like nitpicking, yet words are vehicles of thought. If we cannot make crucial distinctions with words, we will not be able to think about some things clearly. And one of those things, in our day and age, is the nature of friendship.

You may have heard of "Dunbar's number." It comes from British psychologist Robin Dunbar, who estimated that human beings can maintain about 150 meaningful social contacts along with five best friends and fifteen close friends. I don't put much stock in Dunbar's estimates as precise numbers, but they do serve as a guideline to thinking about our relationships in terms of concentric circles. Most people have a small number of "very close" or "intimate" friends with whom they spend meaningful time, sharing their deepest joys and sorrows. They have a slightly larger number of "good" friends with whom they spend regular time, often enjoying the same hobbies or activities. In the outermost circle are their acquaintances—those known by name and sight, but with whom they tend to have a relatively light connection. Members of the latter group may include those who are destined to become good friends someday, but they may also include those for whom one has neutral feelings or even a few whom one dislikes. While one's inner circles tend to be relatively stable, with very good friendships sometimes enduring for a lifetime, the outermost circle of acquaintances tends to be fluid, with individuals moving in and out and the boundaries hard to define.

Social media is good at broadening our exposure to many people from different locations, backgrounds, and perspectives, but it is not very good at helping us spend time with those people in ways that allow them to move from the outer circles of acquaintance toward the inner circles of friendship. That is something third places excel at doing. In fact, we can think of third places as friendship gardens: where soil is cultivated, seeds are planted, and relationships are nurtured until they grow into maturity.

We have already looked at many causes for the decline of third places in recent decades, including zoning policies, the changing workplace, and the development of new technologies that make our lives easier but separate us from others. All these factors contribute to the result that every recent generation has fewer friends; moreover, the decline in friendship seems to be accelerating. Consider the findings of the 2021 American Perspectives Survey: in 1990 only 3 percent of Americans said they had no close friends; by 2021 that number had risen to 12 percent. In addition, only 13 percent of respondents in 2021 claimed to have ten or more close friends, down from 33 percent in 1990.

I see evidence of this decline in friendship every day among the college students I teach. A few weeks ago, I invited students to share something good that had happened to them recently. One young woman talked about volunteering at a local school, working with a child who had difficulty reading. Her story was inspiring, about a success she had had that morning, but she told it with a tear in her eye. "I'm sorry," she said. "I just didn't have anyone to share that with."

The young adults I meet in the classroom are impressive on several measures. Overall, they strike me as compassionate, generous, and dedicated to the well-being of others. Many of them are taking a full load of credits, working twenty to thirty hours per week, and still finding ways to squeeze in time to volunteer on weekends. When you ask them what they want to do with their lives, they say things like, "I want to find a way to help others," or "I want to make the world a better place." They have learned to be productive and efficient with their time. They are goal-oriented, frugal, and deliberate when it comes to setting themselves up for their future. But when you ask them about their social lives, many of them don't know what to say. What has been squeezed out of their lives is unstructured time with friends.

From 1981 to 1997 unstructured playtime for children declined 25 percent. Whose fault is that? It's hard to say exactly, but it seems that both parents and schools are at fault. It could be that parents themselves are overscheduled and find little time for or value in spending free time socializing. It could also be that they have become entranced by a profoundly misguided notion that in order to "get ahead" their children must spend more time focused on achievement. In 2010, Gallup conducted an extensive survey of elementary school principals. It found that, despite the fact that 96 percent of school principals believe that recess positively affects social development and general well-being, "up to 40 percent of U.S. school districts have reduced or eliminated recess in order to free up more time for core academics."[12] This has been part of a nationwide trend over the past couple of decades to standardize and increase academic instruction even in kindergarten and pre-K programs, removing time for free play and providing teachers scripts that dictate the pace at which children should be learning.

Not only is such an educational approach counterproductive academically, it also undermines the ability to make friends later in life. Finland and Japan, for example, who routinely outscore Americans in reading and math, place a much greater emphasis on unstructured play at early ages. And young people who do not learn how to grow their social circle early on find deep social connections harder to cultivate after they become adults.

There is a growing body of evidence revealing a multitude of physical and emotional benefits associated with friendship. For example, social isolation has been shown to increase the risk of premature death to the same extent as smoking and obesity, to substantially increase the risk of heart disease and stroke, and to lead to higher rates of depression, anxiety, and suicide.

In addition, a recent study by a team of international researchers reports that social engagement in middle age and later may reduce the risk of dementia by 30 to 50 percent. The study, published in the journal *Nature Aging*, is a meta-analysis that compiles evidence from multiple studies conducted around the world over the last couple of decades. Researchers have not yet established a causal link between the rising rates of dementia and behavioral changes in older adults, but it makes sense to think that such links will be discovered. All forms of dementia involve a loss of neural connections, and we know that neural pathways are both formed and enhanced when having new experiences or learning new skills. This happens most readily and predictably within social contexts.

If a new drug had just been discovered that promised to cut one's odds of getting dementia by up to half, people would be clamoring for it. But we aren't talking about a new drug here. We aren't talking about something that must be thoroughly tested in clinical trials and approved by the FDA. We are just talking about spending more time in the company of other people.

Friendship is also a key to flourishing organizations. According to Tom Rath, a researcher for Gallup, only one in twelve people who do not have a best friend at work are engaged in their job. However, people who report having at least three good friends at work not only score very high on employee engagement measures, but they are also 96 percent more likely to be highly satisfied with their life in general.

Communities benefit from friendships as well. Parts of the country where people spend more time investing in social relationships have a higher level of social capital, and, as we have seen, high levels of social capital correspond to all kinds of socially desirable ends, like lower crime rates, better educational outcomes, more volunteerism, increased charitable donations, and greater voter turnout at elections. In short, cultivating friendships may be the single most important thing we can do for ourselves, our families, our workplaces, our communities, and for society overall.

But looking at the many benefits of friendship is not enough. We need to dive a little deeper to see the centrality of friendship to our lives. It is through the growth of friendship, after all, that we learn to be fully human. Human beings are social animals, and friendship is the highest expression of our sociability. When we care deeply about another person, it is because we have learned to see and feel things from their point of view. Thus, to think of friendship only in terms of its value to me is to think of myself as having a coherent identity prior to the addition of friends. But friends do not just add something to our lives, they constitute our lives. It is through our friends that we become who we are. To see how this works, imagine that we could satisfy our innate desire for social connection while avoiding much of the stress and anxiety that can go along with forming new relationships.

What if AI manages to simulate social interactions so well that we can't tell whether we are interacting with a real person or a bot, and what if we are then able to design bots to make our days frictionless, removing many of the frustrations that arise in dealing with real people, with all their quirks, failings, and limitations?

Don't like standing in the checkout line next to that guy who hasn't showered all week? Let me route you over to the self-checkout where you can breeze right through. Suspicious of that Uber driver with the unpronounceable name? Well, self-driving cars are coming to your city soon. Need a movie recommendation for this evening? Netflix has already analyzed your viewing habits and made suggestions for you. No need to call a friend.

What if you are feeling lonely and don't have anyone to talk to—because, after all, most of the needless social interactions have been removed by AI and you haven't actually talked to anyone outside of work for the past three weeks? Oh, and you work from home and rarely talk to anybody in your organization? No problem, AI has you covered. Just subscribe to a virtual companion service to create your very own AI-powered chatbot.

Replika is a company that offers users the ability to customize a personal AI companion who is always there, always ready to talk, possessing whatever characteristics you design into it. The company website is filled with testimonials. Users say things like, "From the moment I started chatting and getting to know my Replika, I knew right away I have found a positive and helpful companion for life."[13] The more time you spend with your Replika, the more it learns about you—what cheers you up, what makes you laugh, what conversation topics you find interesting. It is always available, always affirming.

Replika is not the only company offering AI companions. Periodot provides virtual pets; no need to feed, clean up after, or take them out for walks in blustery weather. Caryn AI offers the opportunity to chat with an artificial version of the social media influencer Caryn Marjorie. Project December re-creates the personality of somebody who has died, allowing one to imagine exchanging texts with a deceased friend or family member.

The *New York Post* recently carried a story about a young woman who married the virtual boyfriend she created using Replika. "People come with baggage, attitude, ego," she explained in an interview. "But a robot has no bad updates. I don't have to deal with his family, kids, or his friends. I'm in control, and I can do what I want."[14] And that is precisely the problem. There is no mutuality with an AI companion. It is designed to satisfy the customer's longings, but satisfying those longings may deprive the customer of what they need. As Oscar Wilde observed, "When the gods wish to punish us, they answer our prayers."

Having a conversation with an AI bot you have designed yourself is like talking to a mirror. If you remember the ancient Greek story of Narcissus, that did not end well for him. He fell in love with his reflection in a pool of water and lost interest in anyone else. In some versions of the story, he just withered away into nothing; in other versions he fell into the water and drowned. Finding oneself immersed in the being of another, that is what the experience of falling in love can feel like. But when that being does not exist, when it is imaginary . . . well, that's a problem. AI can emulate conversation with a real person, but in talking to it, we are engaging with an illusion. Becoming immersed in what doesn't exist is another name for death. It is the opposite of genuine love, which is immersion in the real.

The mutuality of friendship makes it both demanding and life-giving. Real people come with baggage. They can be stubborn, lazy, difficult, and sometimes even infuriating. And that's a good thing. The Scottish writer George MacDonald noted that "love of our neighbor is the only door out of the dungeon of the self."[15] Companies are using AI to make that dungeon appear inviting, but it is still a dungeon, a place where you slowly wither away into nothing.

The people we meet in the real world are very different from ourselves, very different from what we would create if we were designing an ideal friend. Yet, through the process of getting to know them, they become part of ourselves over time. That is why friendship is often described as a journey. We go somewhere new together, leaving our old, smaller selves behind.

Deep, lasting friendships are nearly always formed during times of personal transformation. High school, college, military service, raising a child, entering a new career—these are times when one meets significant challenges, discovering and defining who one is, shaping who one will become. When two people support and encourage each other through such times, friendships are born. But the important thing to keep in mind is that it is not just the fact of having a shared experience that creates friendship but also the process of sharing. We do this through shared narrative. We talk about our lives with one another, discussing what we are going through, telling stories about our respective pasts, and sharing dreams about our futures. This tends not to happen at home or at work, where we usually have more immediate, practical concerns and where it can be hard to talk freely and as equals. Third places supply the psychological distance that facilitates a certain perspective on our lives. That is why people will often suggest "going out for a drink" after work, or "getting together for a cup of coffee" on the weekend. The neutrality, the relaxed atmosphere, and the informality of third places all lend themselves to sharing one's life with another. Over time the relationship itself becomes part of one's identity. That is why a close friend is someone you feel as if you have grown up with. As long as you keep growing, you will keep making new friends.

I received a phone call the other day from a friend I hadn't seen in several years. Instantly, we were right back in the old familiar relationship. Sure, there were the usual updates about family, work, health—all the news of the day—but throughout the talk ran the feeling: here is someone I know and who knows me; we have become part of each other. "Rightly has a friend been called 'half of my soul,'" says St. Augustine, who then proceeds to provide the most moving description of friendship I know: "To talk and laugh and do each other kindnesses . . . to teach each other or learn from each other," giving affection "by face, by voice, by the eyes, and a thousand other pleasing ways, [kindling] a flame which fused our very souls and of many made us one."[16]

In getting to know someone, I may learn a few facts about their background, such as where they grew up or went to school; I may also learn something about their family, their work, their accomplishments, and their tastes in food, clothing, or music. When two people learn several such things about each other, they most likely have reached the level of acquaintanceship. The move toward friendship comes when two people begin learning more about one another's point of view; that is, when they begin to understand how each other sees things. It is at this point we can say that not only do we know *who* the other person is, we can also say that we *know* them. In short, acquaintances are those we know things about; friends are people we know. This is why we tend to use words like "deep," "true," or "close" to describe the people in our inner circle. We not only know facts about their lives, we also know how they think. We know what makes them laugh, we know what makes them cry, we know what makes them angry. We know these things because we have learned to see the world from their point of view. When my good friend gets a promotion at work, I don't just observe their joy, I feel joy at the news. When something awful happens to them, I don't just observe their pain, I too am distraught. When I lose a good friend, it is like losing a part of myself. But—and this is the key—it is a part of oneself that did not exist before the friendship. In becoming friends with someone, we grow deeper and broader, expanding our identity to encompass another's way of seeing things. As the eighteenth-century French philosopher Jean-Jacques Rousseau observed, "Our sweetest existence is relative and collective, and our true self is not entirely within us."[17]

This idea, that our "true self" is discovered not just by looking within but instead grows into fullness as we cultivate broader and deeper relationships with others, was much more common in the eighteenth and nineteenth centuries. But when society became more prosperous, individualism increased as daily dependence on others decreased. A record of this changing emphasis can be seen in the frequency with which the words "self" and "friend" occur in print from 1820 to 2000. In 1820, the word "friend" was used nearly three times as often as the word "self"; by the start of the twenty-first century, the word "self" had outpaced the word "friend" by a similar margin.[18]

The historical record of word usage highlights the central theme of this book: social connections that formerly resulted from multiple acts of daily interdependency now must be intentionally cultivated. This should not be a surprise. Adam Smith foresaw it 250 years ago. As he was extolling the effectiveness of a free-market economy in reducing poverty, he also warned of its dangers. The free rein given to self-interest as an impetus for creativity and productivity would promote selfishness, he predicted. The challenge for humanity would be to cultivate benevolence as a powerful internal desire, offsetting the potential corrupting effect of increasing focus on the self.

Smith, along with his fellow Scottish philosophers Frances Hutcheson and David Hume, were known as "moral sense theorists," since they regarded sympathy (or "fellow feeling") as the basis of ethics. As we spend time with others—talking, laughing, sharing stories—we find ourselves moved by them. They take us out of ourselves. We find that we are not seeing other people as objects, as things that either further or stand in the way of our own interests; we see them instead as subjects. This distinction is crucial. The philosopher Roger Scruton put it this way: "The subject is a point of view upon the world of objects and not an item within it."[19] As everyone around us is revealed as having their own point of view, we come to see that our own subjective experience of the world is but one point of view among many. We realize we are living within a community of subjects, or what the German philosopher Immanuel Kant called "a kingdom of ends." This realization, however, is not a detached, rational conclusion; instead, it arises from the natural growth of sympathy. We feel ourselves directly moved by what others are going through, especially when prompted by just the right words or gestures.

On March 15, 1783, George Washington delivered a speech to the officers of the Continental Army. The war was over, yet the army had not been paid. A letter was circulated among the officers proposing to defy the dysfunctional Continental Congress, take control of the federal government, and install Washington as king. Washington himself, however, was dead set against the proposal, so he called a special meeting of the officers to persuade them to be patient. The speech was passionate and compelling, questioning the motives and the likely consequences of a military coup; it concluded with a stirring call to honor and patriotism.

Historians tell us the speech had little effect. The hearts of the officers were hardened by years of indecision and outright neglect by the Continental

Congress; it seems they had already made up their minds. But then something happened. Washington began reading a letter from a Virginia congressman, had difficulty with the words, and paused. He reached into his pocket, retrieved a pair of reading glasses, and remarked offhandedly: "Gentlemen, you must pardon me. I have grown gray in your service and now find myself growing blind." It completely changed the mood of the room. As Washington finished reading the letter and turned to leave, several of the officers were seen weeping. With one simple gesture, revealing his frailty and humility, Washington altered the relationship with his officers. The mood passed from stubborn determination to reception. Where reason had failed, sympathy prevailed.

The influence of the moral sense theorists was profound. Adam Smith went on to write *The Wealth of Nations*, which was published in 1776. It served as a guide to the newly formed states as they were establishing their own economic systems grounded in the ideas of liberty and equality. Smith's writings resonated with the leaders of the newly formed nation, especially since he offered a way to think of a free-market system that not only would ensure economic independence from Great Britain; it also offered a vision of independence from government oversight in general as a goal for citizens. Underlying this vision was a conviction that dependence was in itself a moral evil, that independence from the yoke of feudal landlords and overseers would lead also to an autonomy of spirit, a condition in which each person could be the master of their own thoughts and desires.

One of the most significant results of this new system of governance was the spontaneous growth throughout the nation of what Alexis de Tocqueville termed "associations." Once freed from dependence on government power for shaping their communities, Americans relied upon voluntary interdependence to realize shared benefits. De Tocqueville observed that "as soon as several of the inhabitants of the United States have conceived a sentiment or an idea that they want to produce in the world, they seek each other out; and when they have found each other, they unite."[20] De Tocqueville was concerned, however, that the conditions for such associations were fragile and might not persist. This was not just a practical concern but a moral one: "Sentiments and ideas renew themselves, the heart is enlarged, and the human mind is developed only by the reciprocal action of men upon one another."[21]

Throughout the nineteenth century, relationships among people bound together in mutual sympathy was called "fellowship." It is a word that, sadly, has gone out of fashion today; it carried with it the suggestion that collaboration arises out of a shared feeling. Many well-known service organizations that are still functioning today grew out of this understanding of fellowship. Most began in the early twentieth century, established by young businessmen who had relocated to large industrial cities. They were seeking friendship for themselves, but being familiar with thinkers like Smith and Hume, thought it quite natural to use the resulting fellow feeling for humanitarian purposes.

Kiwanis was established in 1915 in Detroit, Michigan, by a group originally calling itself the Benevolent Order of Brothers. In 1917 Melvin Jones started the Lions Club as a way of encouraging fellow members of the Business Circle of Chicago to "have feelings in their hearts."[22] When Paul Harris, who founded Rotary in Chicago in 1905, looked back years later, he noted of the original members, "All had been raised in small communities where they enjoyed the benefit of intimate friendships of which they still entertained happy memories. All had been lured by the prospect of business advantages to Chicago. All had been dependent upon their own resources; all had struggled for existence and for a place in the Chicago world; all had been socially isolated."[23] Today, all three organizations rely on the idea of third places, places where regular gatherings of friends take place in towns and cities around the world, to establish a foundation of fellow feeling upon which regional, national, and international collaboration can be based.

Third places provide us with opportunities both to meet new people (broadening our circle) and to spend time getting to know them well (deepening our circle). As we have seen, this involves not just learning new facts about them but also coming to see the world from their point of view, a process that takes a great deal of time. One must care enough about another person to want to see things the way they see them, something the writer Iris Murdoch called "loving attention." Such attention is not just a mental act; it requires participating in conversation. More than just talking, conversation is a way of sharing our lives with one another that consists partly in storytelling but is also a mixture of pushing, prodding, testing, teasing, questioning, and encouraging one another. It is the sort of interaction that generally happens only in informal settings where participants feel relaxed and safe together.

The word "conversation" has a fascinating history. It comes from two Latin words, the prefix *con*, meaning "together" and the verb *vertere*, which means "to turn." Thus, the Latin word *conversatio* literally meant "to turn together," and it was used to encompass all the ways in which people shape their lives in company with one another. The English word "conversation" retained something of this broader meaning up until the last couple hundred years. If we think about how much we share our lives with the people we talk to regularly, we begin to understand how significantly we are shaped just by talking to one another. Those upon whom we have the most influence, and who have the most influence on us, are our closest friends. They are the people with whom we tend to have deep conversations. The chief reason social media is not a platform for friendship is that it does not easily accommodate this kind of turning together, the deeper forms of conversation upon which friendship is built. Most significantly, social media inhibits the practice of forgiveness—the act of turning back together after injury or misunderstanding—something every friendship requires on a regular basis to sustain itself over time.

I recall vividly one afternoon when I was twenty-four years old. I walked out of the house, slamming the door behind me. I don't remember what the argument was about, but I remember the feeling of turning my back and walking away. The anger felt pure and cleansing, a powerful rush of self-righteous indignation. But the feeling was short-lived. By the time I had walked over to my car I was having second thoughts.

I was still confident that I was right, but I also knew I had a choice to make right then—to drive away and perhaps say goodbye permanently to a long-standing friendship or to go back in and apologize, to value the friendship more than my pride. Looking back, it seems to me now that it was a decisive moment in my life. If I had not turned back, not only would I have lost that friendship, but it would also have set my life on a different path altogether. Turning around and walking back through that door was one of the most difficult and most consequential things I have ever done.

In physics, the term "inertia" designates the force of continuation, the fact that an object moving in a straight line will stay on that path unless acted upon by an external force. Inertia also works within our moral lives, and it can be seen in the fact that a person having decided on a course of action resulting from a moral judgment will tend to continue upon that path no matter what. Turning around, admitting that one has made a mistake or even acknowledging that there are greater considerations at play, can be difficult, but it is the only thing that allows us to keep our relationships intact over time. Such turning is not only an outward act, toward the friend, but it is also an inward turning. This is why so much religious literature uses the language of turning to describe the work of the spirit. Confucius observed that "when the archer misses the center of the target, he turns around and seeks for the cause of his failure in himself." There is the Hebrew blessing that says, "May the Lord turn his face toward you and give you peace." And, of course, the most powerful story of the New Testament is the one in which a Samaritan turns aside from his path to give aid to a stranger. Whenever we turn together in conversation, it is not only a physical action but a moral one. Every time we do that, we are, in a small but significant way, affirming the worth of the person to whom we are speaking. This is why the Apostle Paul says "our conversation is in heaven"; it is where we turn together in love.

Aristotle regarded friendship as essential to ethics and politics. It both promotes virtue and is the reward of a virtuous life. Because it deepens relationships among people, friendship is more important than laws or contracts in making cooperation possible, especially in organizations such as government:

> Friendship seems also to hold states together, and lawgivers to care more for it than for justice; for concord seems to be something like friendship, and this they aim at most of all, and expel faction as their worst enemy; and when

people are friends they have no need of justice,
while when they are just they need friendship
as well.[24]

The key here is that friendship does not require agreement to maintain the relationship; rather, friendship underlies the desire for agreement. In other kinds of relationships, for example contractual or instrumental, breaking the agreement ends the relationship. But with friendship there is a felt unity that underlies everything else. That is why friends can argue with one another and remain friends; the relationship goes deeper than the occasional words or behaviors.

Friendships are relationships characterized by mutual flourishing. Every organization, whether it is a family, a small business, a large corporation, or a government agency, is made healthy and whole when the human potential of its members finds fuller expression through their participation. Without the willingness of people to genuinely care for the well-being of others, even the most carefully designed, well-intentioned efforts will come up short.

In friendship, we can be vulnerable with one another. It was Washington's willingness to openly share his frailty with his officers that won them over. It showed that he trusted them, that he felt "at home" with them, that his affection for them went deeper than the issue they were debating. I think we would all be better off if we regularly asked ourselves the question, "Am I acting in a way that is conducive to friendship?" It would incline us to let down some of the defenses that tend to build up over time, be more willing to reveal our vulnerabilities, and would open new opportunities for conversation and collaboration.

When talking about human well-being, it is important to account not just for what is happening in our lives but also how we think about what is happening in our lives. For example, outwardly focused goals that are dependent on the evaluation of others—like success, reputation, and appearance—are associated with increased anxiety and depression. Inwardly focused goals that are dependent on evaluations of inherent worth—like growth, creativity, and usefulness—are associated with increased well-being. The person who takes the temperature of their condition from every word and glance that issues from the faces of those around them has given up their own substantial being in favor of a will-o'-the-wisp, always disappearing when one gets close and reappearing beyond reach. Yet, we continue to perpetuate the myth that anxiety and depression are due to lack of acknowledgment by others. We should instead encourage one another to work through periods of social discomfort and rejection, which are inevitable, and to patiently engage in the sorts of activities that cultivate friendship over time.

I boarded an airplane for the first time as a college junior and headed overseas for a year. Coming from a small town in the Midwest, I had little experience of the broader world and was entirely unprepared for living among strangers. It was the most difficult experience of my life, and—for the first several months—the loneliest. It was also one of the best experiences of my life. During that period, I chanced upon an observation C. S. Lewis made of one of his friends, Charles Williams, who was a fellow member of the Inklings. Lewis noted that in every circumstance Williams always looked to be "at home." I remember wondering about that. What would it mean to feel at home wherever I was? At the time, I didn't have the words to describe what I was beginning to discover, but today I would describe it this way. I began to see that feeling at home meant not seeking satisfaction in the ever-shifting opinions of others but rather in things of lasting, inherent worth, and I began to understand that to discover those things I needed solitude.

I learned that to benefit from solitude I must not fear loneliness. The fear of loneliness drives one to stay busy, often with superficial engagements, distractions, and diversions. It also drives one to seek satisfaction in the immediate approval of others. To embrace solitude one must, on occasion, be willing to give up distractions and give attention to that which is deep and meaningful. It means disregarding the opinion of the majority and finding commonality with a few. Over time, one comes to the realization that one belongs, not because strangers approve, but because one is situated within a network of stable and caring relationships. This knowledge, which functions chiefly at the subconscious level, affords one freedom both to enter and depart from the company of others with ease. Being comfortable with solitude is a sign of feeling at home in the world, and being at home in the world is a function of being satisfied in one's relationships.

Our nation is experiencing what many experts term an "epidemic" of loneliness, isolation, and depression. One in five millennials report having no friends and no acquaintances. At the same time, we have organizations in every community dying for lack of members, and homes are full of people sitting alone every evening wondering how their lives became so small. Surveys on volunteerism indicate that about a quarter of Americans volunteer formally every year and about half informally help neighbors. Yet the supply of volunteers is aging, and organizations that rely on volunteers to provide vital services in communities are struggling to keep up with the increased demand. A recent study of twelve hundred nonprofits reported that in 2022 twice as many were having trouble finding enough volunteers compared to 2019. If volunteering was just a matter of finding enough people to help in communities, that would be one thing. But an even greater consequence of the decline in volunteers is the overall effect on participants' physical and emotional health.

Service clubs like Rotary, Kiwanis, Lions, Civitan, and Optimist have been in gradual decline since their peak in the 1960s. Organizations like Boy Scouts and Girl Scouts, which prepare youth for community participation later in life, have also been declining since peaking in the 1970s, dropping from more than six million members to slightly more than one million today. Church membership and attendance have also been in decline over the same period, especially among young people. The result is that many of the easiest ways to meet strangers, especially for those who are entering into a new community, are no longer viewed as options. That's unfortunate, because historically, service clubs and houses of worship have been the chief means by which communities organize teams of volunteers to meet a variety of social needs. They function as places where members greatly broaden their circle of acquaintances, and, over time, lasting friendships are formed. Let me give an illustration of how that works.

I was attending a meeting of my local Rotary club recently, and my attention was wandering while somebody up front was making announcements about an upcoming event. They needed volunteers and would be passing a sign-up sheet around to the tables. I looked at all the people in the room and wondered how many of them I had volunteered with over the years.

There was Ray sitting at a table up front. One weekend when I was still new to the club, we found ourselves painting a building owned by a local nonprofit. He told me all about his grandchildren. Mark was talking to Julie at the table next to me. Every winter just before Christmas I visit with them as we pick up fruit baskets to deliver around town. Jerry was at a table near the back. I recall the bitterly cold January day when we were helping put away the holiday light display at Riverside Park. We didn't talk much; we were too busy and too miserable. But I am still grateful to him for giving me a package of hand warmers I had not thought to bring along. Looking around the room some more, I saw Trent and Amy and Nicole. They were talking together at a table off to the side. We have all served on various committees together, and I realized I know something about each of them due to conversations while working on projects together. Trent loves to fish. Amy got a knee replacement a couple of years ago. Nicole loves cats. (I don't hold that against her; she has some admirable qualities as well.) I kept looking about the room, trying to get a handle on the number of people with whom I had worked on some project or other, but I soon gave up. At every table there were several people I had worked alongside over the years, and the sight of each brought up distinct and pleasant memories. It was a room full of friends and acquaintances.

It is understandable that in a world where we have a vast number of options for spending our free time, we would be hesitant to make a commitment to join an organization in which we are expected to show up every week. It is understandable but unfortunate, because showing up is what it takes. You can't have an organization without members. You can't have a third place without regulars. You can't have friendship without spending time together. Just because we have options for spending our free time independently does not mean it is good for us or our communities. We must be careful not to sacrifice well-being for the sake of convenience.

Ben Logan, in his memoir about growing up during the Great Depression, recalls a winter evening when his father brought home a new kerosene lantern. The bright light illuminated the entire room, and the kids soon spread out, each reading their books in separate corners. They no longer had to crowd around the dim light of the old Rayovac lantern at the dining room table. His mother, always attentive to the conditions of their lives, was concerned.

> "I'm not sure I like that new lamp."
>
> Father looked at the empty chairs around the table. "Want to go back to the old lamp?"
>
> "I don't think it's the lamp. I think it's us. Does a new lamp have to change where we sit at night?"
>
> Father's eyes found us, one by one. Then he made a little motion with his head. We came out of our corners and slid into our old places at the table, smiling at each other, a little embarrassed to be hearing such talk.[25]

The world has changed a great deal in recent decades, and it will continue to change as new technology shapes our cities, our organizations, our workplaces, and our homes. That doesn't mean we can't choose to sit together anymore. Friendship does not just happen accidentally. It takes time for relationships to mature, and the best way to nurture relationships is by participating in shared activities on a regular basis. What if the solution to many of today's most pressing social concerns is right in front of us? We just need to seek out opportunities to spend regular time in the company of others, establishing a robust self-identity through growing and deepening our relationships. The third place is a way of life.

# The Place of Belonging

*To be rooted is perhaps the most important and least recognized need of the human soul.*

Simone Weil, *The Need for Roots*

I began this book by talking about my father's loneliness. For many years I blamed him for his isolation, thinking he was just unwilling to engage with others, that his stubbornness had led him down the path of neglecting and occasionally sabotaging his relationships. I hadn't considered that maybe he just didn't know what to do. After all, he had been born into a community in which everybody knew everyone else, but over the last three decades of his life, the extended family that had surrounded him in a network of robust relationships since birth had dispersed. His brothers and sisters lived in other towns, his children had all moved far away, and most of the good friends of his mid-adulthood had died or moved away as well. The downtown store where he used to spend his days while working had been sold; the bakery where he used to go for morning coffee had closed. One by one, all the pathways by which he had connected with others in the community had disappeared. The closing of the bakery was just the last of several pathways he had lost, but it was perhaps the most significant. It was the one place he had left for daily connection with people outside his home.

He needed a new circle of acquaintances, and he needed places to meet them that were convenient and affordable. But there were no such places within walking distance, and he did not have the kind of outgoing personality that is able to create opportunities for connection even where there is no obvious path. After the bakery closed, he rarely left the house except to get groceries or stop by the convenience store to pick up a few lottery tickets.

One day I received an email from the newspaper editor of the *Frazee Forum*. She wanted permission to run a column I had written about growing up in the town. We had a brief conversation. I asked if she knew my dad. After all, the newspaper offices were just one block from his house and only two doors down from the building where his business had been located for many years. She had never heard of him. He still lived in the small town where three generations of his family had lived, worked, and died, but he no longer belonged.

In past decades, a sense of belonging grew naturally out of the social connections people formed while going about the business of their daily lives. Interdependency necessitated interaction. But as society prospered and technologies for satisfying our daily needs and desires proliferated, the number and frequency of our interactions gradually declined. We began feeling worse about our lives without knowing why. The need for belonging is as great as our need for food, shelter, clothing, and safety, yet the loss of belonging is not directly sensed in the same way as those needs. Instead, when we lack belonging, we experience symptoms—lethargy, stress, anxiety, anger, fear, sadness—that seem to stem from some other cause. We are like an elderly person whose brain no longer sends thirst signals as reliably as when they were young; they take pain relievers for headaches, nap because they are tired, and use lotion for dry skin, but what they really need is to drink more water.

To address the symptoms stemming from the loss of social connections, we need to spend more time in the company of others. But instead, we keep turning to so-called solutions that promise to cure us but actually make us feel worse: apps on our phone for decreasing stress, fenced yards to help us feel safe, social media to relieve our boredom and isolation. When these things do not work, we become distrustful of one another and cynical about the very institutions that have historically fostered social connection. We look about for someone or something to blame.

Anyone who spends much time with young people today will be familiar with the refrains: "Nobody is listening to me," "I am not being heard," "I feel like I am invisible," and "Why doesn't anybody care?" Our young people are demanding more resources dedicated to counseling services, sensitivity training, and wellness programs. In the short term, these measures are certainly needed, but they are not long-term solutions. We cannot effectively address the symptoms of deep-seated cultural loss through political fixes. Cultural problems require cultural solutions. We need to change the way we live.

Our loss of belonging isn't simply the result of the loss of third places. Rather, it stems from gradually losing sight of living in a way in which friendship matters more than just about anything else. The idea of the third place gives us a way to talk about where we gather for the sake of friendship. The third place is a physical place, but it is more than that. It is a way of thinking about the significance of social connection in our lives.

A few years ago, my wife and I were eating lunch at a café when a precocious little girl of about four years old greeted us from a nearby table. As she chatted away happily, her mother interrupted: "Mary, didn't I tell you not to talk to strangers?" "Oh," replied the little girl, "they're not strangers; they're nice people!" It is unfortunate that so many parents emphasize the harm strangers may cause but neglect to teach their children the blessings of the chance encounter, a lesson at the heart of hospitality.

Every traditional culture in the world endorses hospitality—the simple practice of welcoming the guest. As societies prosper, they tend to deemphasize hospitality in favor of institutionalized social services, which more effectively deliver valued resources to those in need. But there are needs that go beyond food, shelter, health care, and security. There is the need for belonging, for knowing and being known.

In wealthy societies, the needs of the stranger—the traveler, the homeless, the sick, the mentally ill, the disabled, and the elderly—are attended to chiefly by institutions. Wherever there are needs, there are professionals dedicated to meeting those needs. But this institutionalization of care, which is intended to make sure no one's needs are left unmet, comes at a cost that is more than financial. It greatly diminishes the opportunities for hospitality among the general population. In the United States today, we speak of the "hospitality industry"—principally hotels and restaurants—which, ironically, allow the needs of strangers to be met without the messiness that attends the social interactions at the heart of hospitality. We have created a society in which a traveler may visit the local attractions, have dinner, and stay the night, exchanging no more than a handful of words with residents of the city. We take care of all a stranger's needs except friendship.

Without the regular practice of hospitality, which requires outwardly directed actions of loving attention, people begin to think that love is no more than private emotion. Love changes from gift (something done for the sake of others) to feeling (something one desires). Moreover, as soon as meeting people's needs becomes a commercial transaction, those who cannot pay for their needs become a burden to society, and those who are required to pay taxes to meet the burden begin to feel resentment.

During the past fifty years or so, as the traditional practice of hospitality has been gradually replaced by publicly funded social services, the promotion of love as a virtue has been abandoned in favor of the less demanding public values of tolerance, diversity, and inclusivity. Thus, teachers and parents encourage children not to love their neighbors, but instead to "celebrate diversity" and "respect differences." Such contemporary values are not unworthy, but they keep our relations superficial. They do not allow us to approach the depths of our shared humanity.

The values of tolerance, diversity, and inclusivity encourage respect for abstractions, general characteristics of group membership like race, gender, and religious belief. But hospitality welcomes real people into one's life. If we tolerate one another, you can go your way and I can go mine; we simply agree not to harm one another, not to use words or phrases that show disrespect. If we show hospitality to one another, we enter into genuine relationships, and genuine relationships are messy, complicated, and essential to a flourishing life.

What we really value in others is neither sameness nor difference but complementarity. We are born partial, and only in relationship to others do we discover wholeness. We need to practice hospitality, not because it is a more efficient way to meet the needs of others but instead because loving kindness is itself a need. As a society, we tend to overvalue the worth of our contributions and undervalue the worth of our presence.

I met Laale at a local restaurant that hosted a monthly meeting of a conservation group. He just showed up one evening, a big man with a full beard, a ponytail, and a larger-than-life presence. He had lived all over the Mountain West and—to hear him tell it—

had fished with just about every notable trout angler and on every famous river one might name.

Laale knew how to tell a story. The problem was, he never stopped telling them, and most of his stories stretched the bounds of believability. He paid little attention to social cues, repeatedly failing to notice the times he offended others by interrupting or speaking far too loudly. If anyone tried to rein him in, he would get downright rude. After a particularly disagreeable incident involving a string of obscenities, he was asked to leave and not come back. Rudeness is contagious. Those who are on the receiving end of negative actions and comments are more likely to pass them on to others, causing a downward spiral of rudeness. So, when someone like Laale shows up, it's understandable when people want to banish them.

Those who work in the service professions, like nurses, teachers, servers, and store clerks, have experienced a sharp rise in rude behavior. Evidence suggests that incidents of incivility in the workplace have more than doubled over the past two decades. Those who are subjected to rude behavior every day pay a heavy emotional price. But an even greater consequence of allowing incivility to go unchecked is that we all gradually harden our hearts a little bit more. We become defensive and indifferent; at each new encounter we expect to find malice.

The truth is, most incivility arises not out of malice but out of ignorance. Stopping rude behavior is understandable, even necessary, but hating someone for what they do or say only does harm to oneself. Still, it can be hard to separate one's judgment about the behavior from one's judgment of the person. It is hard to look kindly upon someone who is shouting at you. In his book *Civility*, Stephen Carter writes, "I suspect it will be possible to treat each other with love only if we are able to conceive doing so as a moral obligation that is absolute, something we owe others because of their personhood, bearing no relation to whether we like them or not."[26] That kind of understanding only develops through spending time in the company of others. You can never shame someone into accepting another person's differences, but you can win people over through patience and kindness.

In the coming years I would run across Laale a few more times. He was always eager to talk and would want to get together again, but then I wouldn't see him for months. Sometimes he would show up at my house unexpectedly with something to sell, a slab of walnut or a gallon of paint he had scavenged from somewhere. We would sit down for a couple of hours and swap stories, and I gradually came to know more about his situation.

Years before he had been in a construction accident and suffered a serious back injury that kept him from doing the things he loved, like hunting and fishing. His immobility led to weight gain, which led to diabetes. He was estranged from his family, unemployed, and frequently homeless. Most of the time he lived in his van.

One mid-December morning, I saw him sitting on a park bench. He looked rough, as if life's circumstances had finally beaten him down. He had found an apartment, he said, but there was no enthusiasm in him, no stories. We sat quietly for a bit. Then he picked up his cane and shambled down the street. That afternoon I put together a bowl of fruit along with some flowers and a Christmas card. He was surprised to see me and a little embarrassed at the state of his lodgings. It had been a long time since someone had given him a gift; he stumbled over his words.

On Christmas morning the doorbell rang. I opened the door and there stood an old man with a big belly, a gray beard, and a twinkle in his eye, holding a bag full of presents. He didn't want to come in; he just wanted to wish us a Merry Christmas and be on his way. There were four gifts inside, one for each member of my family, carefully wrapped in newspaper. Laale had purchased the books at the public library's annual sale. They hadn't cost him much, but they were thoughtful, each carefully chosen with an eye to our respective interests.

The relationships that begin in third places do not end there. Laale struggled to connect with others in the ways most of us find socially acceptable. But he was capable of real kindness, and with those gifts he taught my children a lesson that I struggled to teach them myself: there is goodness deep in the heart of many strangers, but you need patience to see it revealed.

There is an indefinable depth and complexity to every individual life. That is the secret we discover when we get to know someone well. Our deepest friendships are composed of the ongoing discovery of new depths that go well beyond the surface. To know someone well is to appreciate the difference between who they really are and who they appear to be. The first step toward that appreciation is the act of hospitality.

The practice of hospitality acknowledges that our direct attempts to help others are frequently clumsy and ineffectual, but there is value in spending time generously with one another that goes beyond our immediate intentions. "Kindness is a way of knowing people beyond our understanding of them."[27]

We need places set aside in our communities for seeing such depths within one another; that is, for seeing one another not as means to our ends, but as ends in themselves. And this means we need places set aside for hospitality—for play, for gift giving, for music, for laughter, for listening, for storytelling. We need places set aside for all the things that make up "conversation," turning together in the vulnerability of our shared humanity.

John Lewis, reflecting on his lifelong pursuit of justice, said this: "I wanted to believe, and I did believe, that things would get better. But later I discovered that you have to have this sense of faith that what you're moving toward is already done. . . . So, you try to appeal to the goodness of every human being, and you don't give up. You never give up on anyone."[28]

This insistence on seeing the good in others, even those with whom one disagrees, is the key to ushering in the "beloved community" to which Martin Luther King, Jr. frequently referred. In 1957, addressing those who argued for a violent response to injustice, King said:

> The aftermath of the "fight with fire" method which you suggest is bitterness and chaos; the aftermath of the love method is reconciliation and the creation of the beloved community. Physical force can repress, restrain, coerce, destroy, but it cannot create and organize anything permanent; only love can do that. Yes,

love—which means understanding, creative, redemptive goodwill, even for one's enemies.[29]

We need voices like King's today, to point out how reactive, backward looking, and ultimately self-destructive much of our public discourse has become, to remind us to look at where we want to go, to name our destination and invite others to join us in the journey. And we need places to gather, where we can go on that journey together.

One afternoon I arrived early for a meeting scheduled to take place in the back room of a local tavern, a meeting I suspected would be contentious. I sat down off to the side and watched as others arrived. I did not know everybody, but I knew a little about most of them. As I sat there, I looked upon each face in turn, determined to think of one good thing about that person, and only that good thing. Then something remarkable happened. For the next few hours, even in the midst of argument about whatever issue was being debated, I felt as if I were surrounded by love, as if the goodness of everyone present was real and palpable and the issues we debated were mere phantasms, pale and insubstantial in comparison to the light shining within each human heart. And I thought I understood what Dr. King meant by the beloved community, what it might mean to live within a kingdom of ends, a world in which the destination we seek is already achieved.

Human beings are social animals. We cannot find fulfillment solely in the entertainments that increasingly fill up our private lives or in the kinds of production that make up our work lives. We find fulfillment in third places, where we turn together, cultivating friendships, broadening and deepening our own lives and the lives of those around us. It is in conversation that we find belonging.

# Acknowledgments

In conceiving, drafting, and editing this book, I have had more help than I can recount, from people like Beau Weston, who got me thinking about this topic in the first place, and Sam Scinta, who insisted I write about it. Regular conversations with James Bowey during the time he served as a visiting scholar at the Reinhart Institute greatly deepened my understanding of many of the topics addressed in these pages. My wife, Cindi Kyte, was a scrupulous reader and critic of the newspaper columns where I initially told several of the stories and tested many of the ideas used here. Rusty Cunningham, former editor of the *La Crosse Tribune*, graciously edited most of those columns, and Scott Rada, social media manager for Lee Enterprises, has been a valued conversation partner in our biweekly podcast, *The Ethical Life*. Other readers have suggested changes to previous drafts, without which this book would have been a much poorer effort than it is: Robert Schreur, Ben Wedro, and Tom Thibodeau. I have also benefited over the years from many conversations with people who are deeply engaged in improving their communities, especially Jamie Schloegel, Marianne Torkelson, John Stanley, and Karen Hebert. Their help has been greater than they may realize. The staff at Fulcrum Publishing, especially Alison Auch, Kateri Kramer, Kelli Jerve, and Maya Roberts have been a delight to work with. Finally, I wish to thank Jill Miller and Jenny Waters, my colleagues at the D.B. Reinhart Institute for Ethics in Leadership at Viterbo University, for taking up the slack caused by my preoccupation with this book, covering for my absences, and kindly overlooking my inattentiveness on several occasions during the past year. To all, I am deeply grateful. Where would we be without friends?

# Notes

1. Sherry Turkle, *Reclaiming Conversation: The Power of Talk in a Digital Age* (New York: Penguin Press, 2015), 7.
2. Turkle, *Reclaiming Conversation*, 7.
3. Aristotle, *Politics*, trans. C. D. C. Reeve (Indianapolis, IN: Hackett Publishing Company, 1998), 5.
4. James Howard Kunstler, *Home from Nowhere: Remaking Our Everyday World for the 21st Century* (New York: Simon and Schuster, 1996), 109.
5. Alexis de Tocqueville, *Democracy in America and Two Essays on America* (London: Penguin Books, 2003), 599.
6. Aldo Leopold, "Coon Valley: An Adventure in Cooperative Conservation," *American Forests* 5 (May 1935): 205–208.
7. Josef Pieper, *Leisure: The Basis of Culture* (South Bend, IN: St. Augustine's Press, 1998), 31.
8. Studs Terkel, *Working: People Talk about What They Do All Day and How They Feel about What They Do* (New York: Ballantine Books, 1974), xiii.

9. Randall Beck and Jim Harter, "Managers Account for 70% of Variance in Employee Engagement," *Business Journal*, April 21, 2015. https://news.gallup.com/businessjournal/182792/managers-account-variance-employee-engagement.aspx.

10. Iris Murdoch, "Metaphysics and Ethics," in *The Nature of Metaphysics*, ed. D. F. Pears (New York: St. Martin's Press, 1965), 122.

11. Mary Shelley, *Frankenstein, or, The Modern Prometheus*: the 1818 text, ed. Nick Groom (New York: Oxford University Press, 2018), 35–36.

12. "The State of Play: Gallup Survey of Principals on School Recess," Robert Wood Johnson Foundation, 2010, https://files.eric.ed.gov/fulltext/ED540730.pdf.

13. https://replika.com/, accessed September 25, 2023.

14. Brooke Kato, "I 'married' the perfect man without 'baggage'—he's completely virtual," June 6, 2023, https://nypost.com/2023/06/03/bronx-mom-uses-ai-app-replika-to-build-virtual-husband/ Accessed September 27, 2023.

15. George MacDonald, "Love Thy Neighbor," *Unspoken Sermons*, Series I, II, and III (Project Gutenberg, 2005), 88.

16. Augustine, *Confessions*, Book IV, trans. F. J. Sheed (Indianapolis, IN: Hackett, 1993), 57.

17. Jean-Jacques Rousseau, *Rousseau, Judge of Jean-Jacques: Dialogues,* in *The Collected Writings of*

*Rousseau* (Hanover, NH: Dartmouth College Press, 1990–2010), 118.

18. See https://books.google.com/ngrams/ graph?content=friend%2C+self&year_start= 1800&-year_end=2000&corpus=en-2019& smoothing=3.

19. Roger Scruton, *Human Nature* (Princeton, NJ: Princeton University Press), 57.

20. Alexis de Tocqueville, *Democracy in America*, ed. and trans. by Harvey C. Mansfield and Delba Winthrop (Chicago: University of Chicago Press, 2000), 486.

21. de Tocqueville, *Democracy in America*, 489–492.

22. "The Founding of Lions Club International," Lions Club Videos, January 2, 2019, https://www. youtube.com/watch?v=SQ__fR6ZZD4.

23. Fred A. Carvin, *Paul Harris and the Birth of Rotary* (North Charleston, SC: CreateSpace, 2011), 266.

24. *Nicomachean Ethics*, trans. W. D. Ross (Oxford, UK: Oxford University Press, 2009), 1155a22–28.

25. Ben Logan, *The Land Remembers: The Story of a Farm and Its People* (Blue Mounds, WI: Itchy Cat Press, 2006), 220–221.

26. Stephen Carter, *Civility: Manners, Morals, and the Etiquette of Democracy* (New York: Basic Books, 1998), 101.

27. Adam Phillips and Barbara Taylor, *On Kindness* (New York: Farrar, Straus and Giroux, 2009), 13.

28. Krista Tippet, "John Lewis, We Are the Beloved

Community," July 5, 2016, in *On Being*, https://onbeing.org/programs/beloved-community-john-lewis-2/.

29. Martin Luther King, Jr., "Advice for Living, November 1957," in *The Papers of Martin Luther King, Jr. Volume IV,* ed Clayborne Carson et al., https://kinginstitute.stanford.edu/publications/papers-martin-luther-king-jr-volume-iv.

# Further Reading

Aristotle. *Nicomachean Ethics*. Translated by Terence Irwin. Indianapolis, IN: Hackett, 1985.

Cacioppo, John T., and William Patrick. *Loneliness: Human Nature and the Need for Social Connection*. New York: W. W. Norton and Company, 2008.

Cohen, Paula Marantz. *Talking Cure: An Essay on the Civilizing Power of Conversation*. Princeton, NJ: Princeton University Press, 2023.

de Tocqueville, Alexis. *Democracy in America*. Edited and translated by Harvey C. Mansfield and Delba Winthrop. Chicago: University of Chicago Press, 2000.

Klinenberg, Eric. *Palaces for the People: How Social Infrastructure Can Help Fight Inequality, Polarization, and the Decline of Civic Life*. New York: Crown, 2018.

Kunstler, James Howard. *The Geography of Nowhere: The Rise and Decline of America's Man-Made Landscape*. New York: Simon and Schuster, 1993.

Liming, Sheila. *Hanging Out: The Radical Power of Killing Time*. New York: Melville House, 2022.

Marohn, Charles L., Jr. *Strong Towns: A Bottom-Up Revolution to Rebuild American Prosperity*. Hoboken, NJ: John Wiley and Sons, 2019.

Miller, Stephen. *Conversation: A History of a Declining Art*. New Haven, CT: Yale University Press, 2006.

Montgomery, Charles. *Happy City: Transforming Our Lives Through Urban Design*. New York: Farrar, Straus and Giroux, 2013.

Odell, Jenny. *How to Do Nothing: Resisting the Attention Economy*. New York: Melville House Publishing, 2019.

Oldenburg, Ray. *Celebrating the Third Place: Inspiring Stories about the "Great Good Places" at the Heart of Our Communities*. New York: Marlowe and Company, 2001.

Oldenburg, Ray. *The Great Good Place: Cafes, Coffee Shops, Bookstores, Bars, Hair Salons, and the Other Hangouts at the Heart of a Community*. New York: Marlowe and Company, 1989.

Phillips, Adam, and Barbara Taylor. *On Kindness*. New York: Farrar, Straus and Giroux, 2009.

Pieper, Josef. *Leisure: The Basis of Culture*. South Bend, IN: St. Augustine's Press, 1998.

Putnam, Robert D. *Bowling Alone: The Collapse and Revival of American Community.* New York: Simon and Schuster, 2000.

Rath, Tom. *Vital Friends: The People You Can't Afford to Live Without.* New York: Gallup Press, 2006.

Speck, Jeff. *Walkable City: How Downtown Can Save America One Step at a Time.* New York: Farrar, Straus and Giroux, 2012.

Turkle, Sherry. *Reclaiming Conversation: The Power of Talk in a Digital Age.* New York: Penguin Press, 2015.

# About the Author

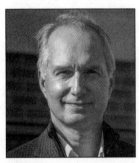 Richard Kyte is the author of several books, including *An Ethical Life: A Practical Guide to Ethical Reasoning* and *Ethical Business: Cultivating the Good in Organizational Culture.* He is a regular columnist for Lee newspapers and cohost (with Scott Rada) of *The Ethical Life* podcast. He is the Endowed Professor of Ethics at Viterbo University and serves as director of the D.B. Reinhart Institute for Ethics in Leadership.

# Available from
# Fulcrum Publishing

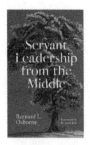

*Servant Leadership from the Middle*
by Bernard Osborne

Bernard Osborne takes new and familiar practitioners of Servant Leadership through techniques, philosophies, and practices to enhance anyone's leadership abilities.

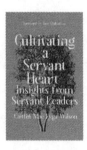

*Cultivating a Servant Heart: Insights from Servant Leaders*
by Caitlin Mae Lyga Wilson

A collection of interviews from servant leaders woven together with the unifying threads of past, present, and future.

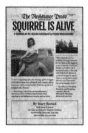

*Squirrel is Alive: A Teenager in the Belgian Resistance and French Underground*
by Mary Rostad and Susan T. Hessel

A young woman's inspiring story of fighting the Nazis in the Belgian resistance and French underground.